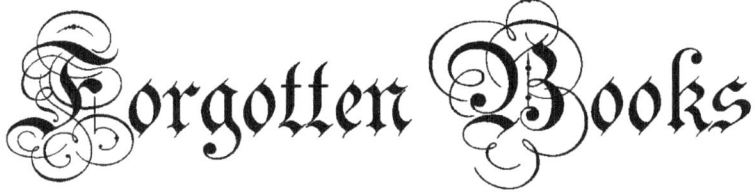
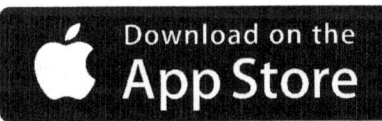
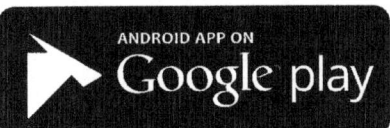

ISBN 978-1-331-08543-0
PIBN 10142905

1 MONTH OF
FREE
READING

at

www.ForgottenBooks.com

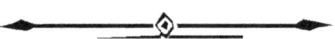

By purchasing this book you are eligible for one month membership to ForgottenBooks.com, giving you unlimited access to our entire collection of over 700,000 titles via our web site and mobile apps.

To claim your free month visit:

www.forgottenbooks.com/free142905

Similar Books Are Available from
www.forgottenbooks.com

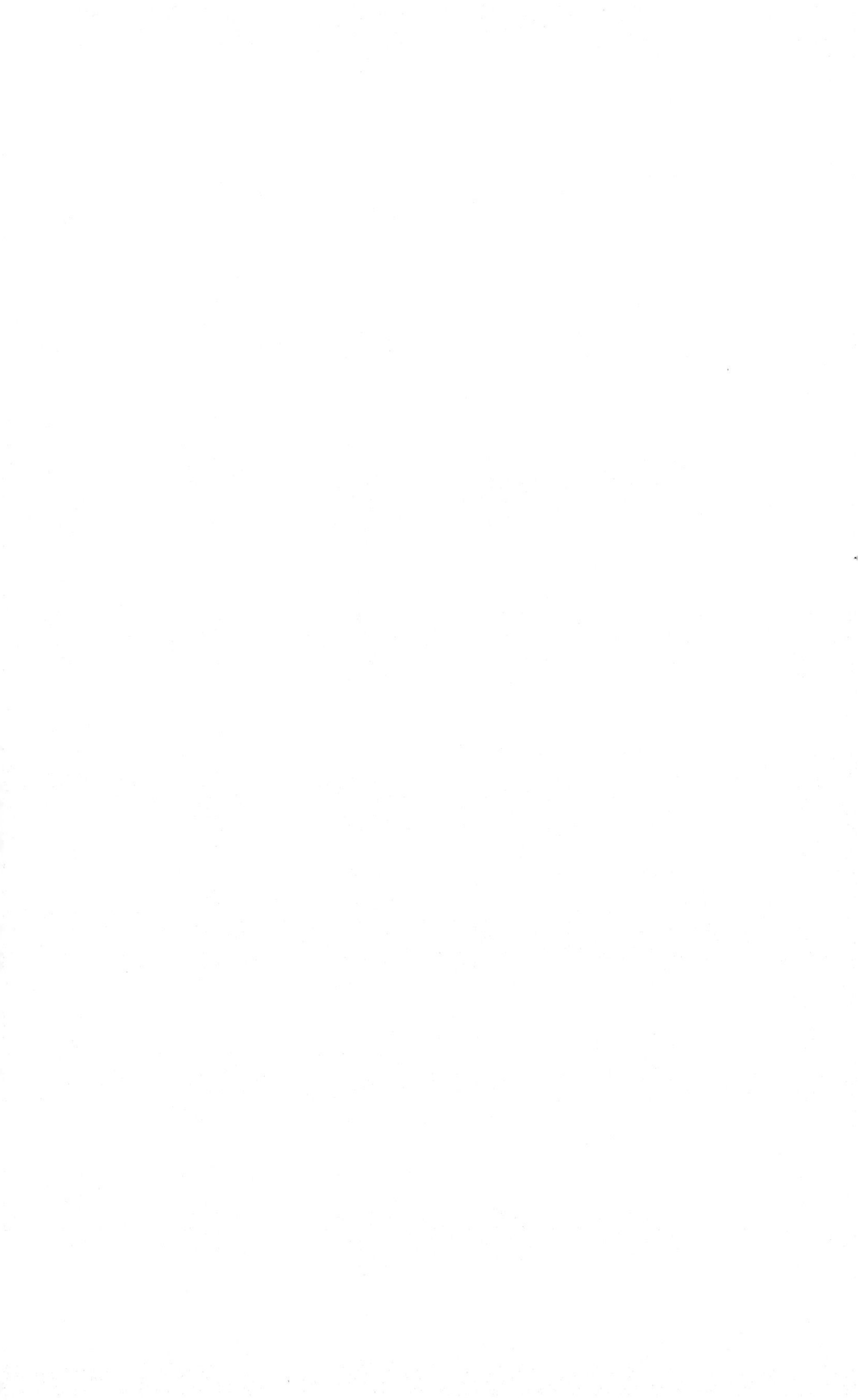

LECTURES

ON

DISEASES OF THE NERVOUS SYSTEM,

ESPECIALLY IN WOMEN.

BY

S. WEIR MITCHELL, M.D.,

MEMBER OF THE NATIONAL ACADEMY OF SCIENCES;
PHYSICIAN TO THE ORTHOPÆDIC HOSPITAL, AND INFIRMARY FOR DISEASES OF THE
NERVOUS SYSTEM;
FELLOW OF THE PHILADELPHIA COLLEGE OF PHYSICIANS;
MEMBER OF THE NEW YORK ACADEMY OF MEDICINE;
ASSOCIATE FELLOW OF THE AMERICAN ACADEMY OF ARTS AND SCIENCES OF BOSTON;
HONORARY MEMBER OF THE STATE MEDICAL SOCIETIES OF NEW YORK,
NEW JERSEY, AND MARYLAND;
HONORARY CORRESPONDING MEMBER OF THE BRITISH MEDICAL ASSOCIATION;
HONORARY FELLOW OF THE LONDON MEDICAL SOCIETY;
HONORARY MEMBER OF THE ST. ANDREW'S MEDICAL GRADUATES' ASSOCIATION;
FOREIGN ASSOCIATE OF THE ROYAL MEDICAL SOCIETY OF NORWAY ·
AUTHOR OF A TREATISE ON INJURIES OF NERVES, ETC. ETC.

WITH FIVE PLATES.

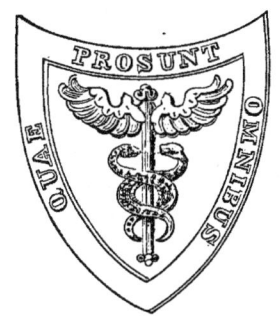

PHILADELPHIA:
HENRY C. LEA'S SON & CO.
1881.

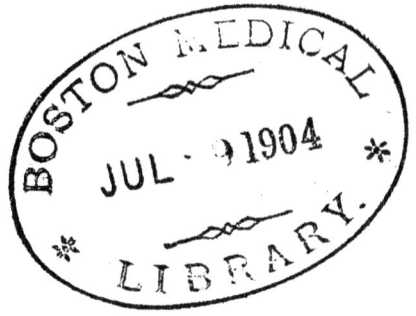

COLLINS, PRINTER.

DEDICATED TO

J. HUGHLINGS–JACKSON, M.D., F.R.S.,

WITH WARM PERSONAL REGARD,

AND

IN GRATEFUL ACKNOWLEDGMENT

OF

HIS SERVICES TO

THE SCIENCE OF MEDICINE.

PREFACE.

THE lectures which compose this volume deal chiefly with some of the rarer maladies, or forms of maladies, of women. Many of them are original studies of well-known diseases, and others deal with subjects which have been hitherto slighted in medical literature or which are almost unknown to it.

I desire to express my thanks for very valuable aid to my colleague Dr. WHARTON SINKLER, to Professor HORATIO C. WOOD, to Dr. LOUIS STARR, and especially to Dr. MORRIS J. LEWIS.

CONTENTS

LECTURE I.

THE PARALYSES OF HYSTERIA.

LECTURE II.

HYSTERICAL MOTOR ATAXIA—HYSTERICAL PARESIS.

LECTURE III.

MIMICRY OF DISEASE.

LECTURE IV.

MIMICRY OF DISEASE.

LECTURE V.

UNUSUAL FORMS OF SPASMODIC AFFECTIONS IN WOMEN.

LECTURE VI.

TREMOR—CHRONIC SPASMS.

LECTURE VII.

CHOREA OF CHILDHOOD.

LECTURE VIII.

HABIT CHOREA.

LECTURE XIII.

For Description of Plates, with Remarks, see
pages 127 to 145.

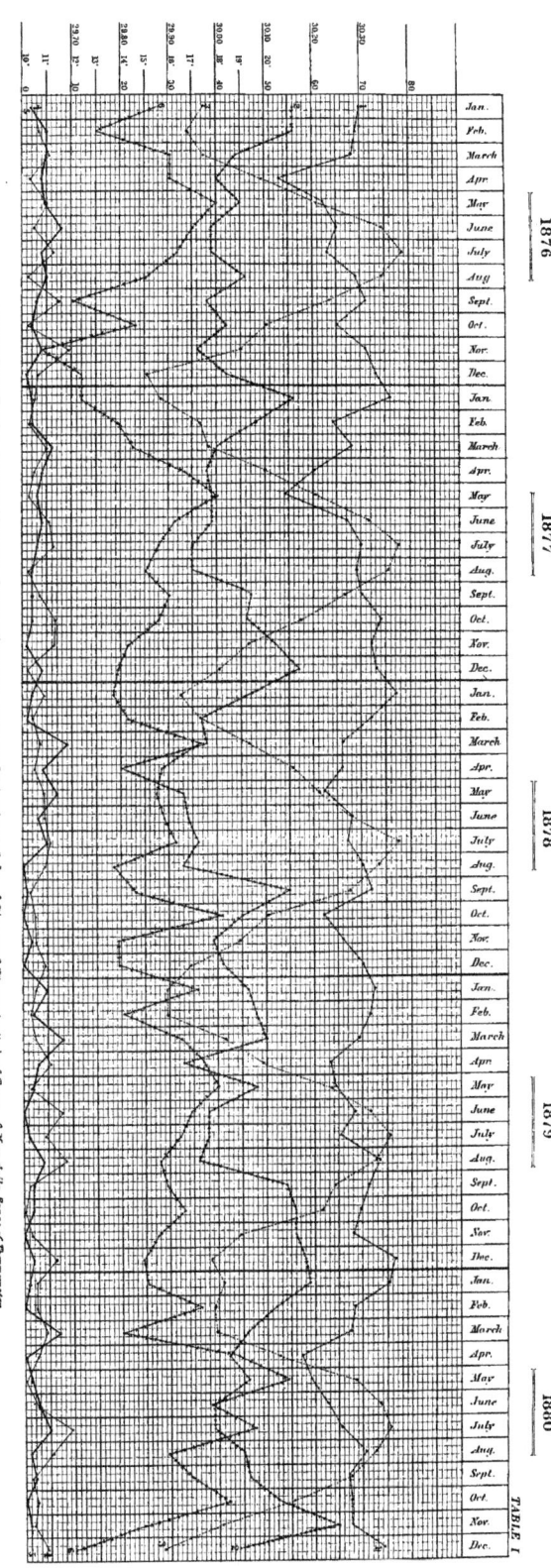

1876 1877 1878 1879 1880 TABLE I.

1 Average Relative Humidity. 2 Average of Barometer. 3 Average Temperature. 4 Amount of Rain & Snow in Inches 5 Diagram of 191 separate strains of Cholera 6 Mean daily Range of Thermometer.

80

30,30   70

30.20   60

30.10 20° 50

19°

30.00 18°

17°

29.90 16°

15°

29.80 14°

13°

29.70 12°

11°

10°

1. *Average Relative Humidity*
2. *Average of Barometer*
3. *Average Temperature*
4. *Amount of Rain & Snow in inches*
5. *Diagram of 170 separate attacks of Chorea*
6. *Mean daily Range of Thermometer*

1876 – 80

TABLE III

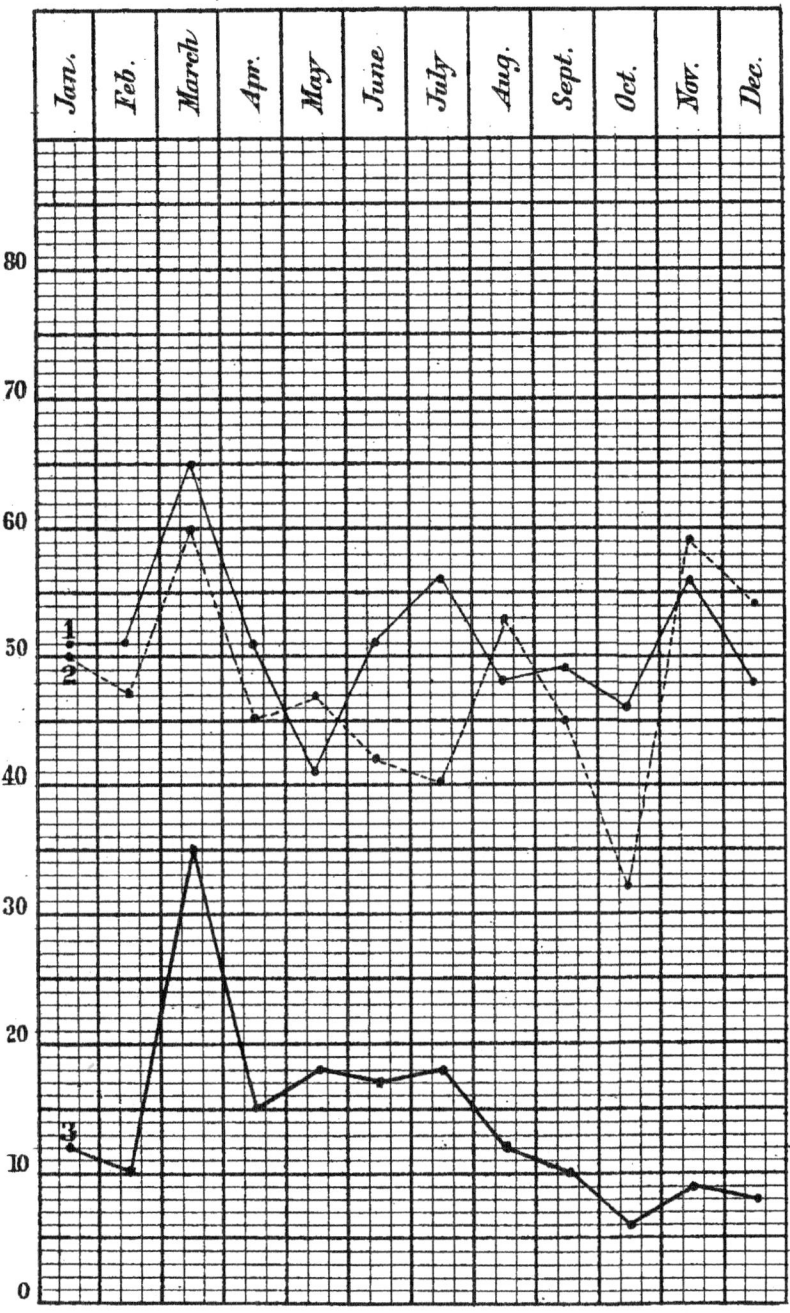

1 No. of Days on which rain or snow fell
2 No of Cloudy days
3 No. of separate attacks of Chorea

1878-80

TABLE IV

1 No of Storms centers passing within 150 Miles of Phila
2 „ „ „ „ „ „ 400 „ „ „
3 No. of separate attacks of Chorea

1871 *to* 1880 *inclusive*

TABLE V

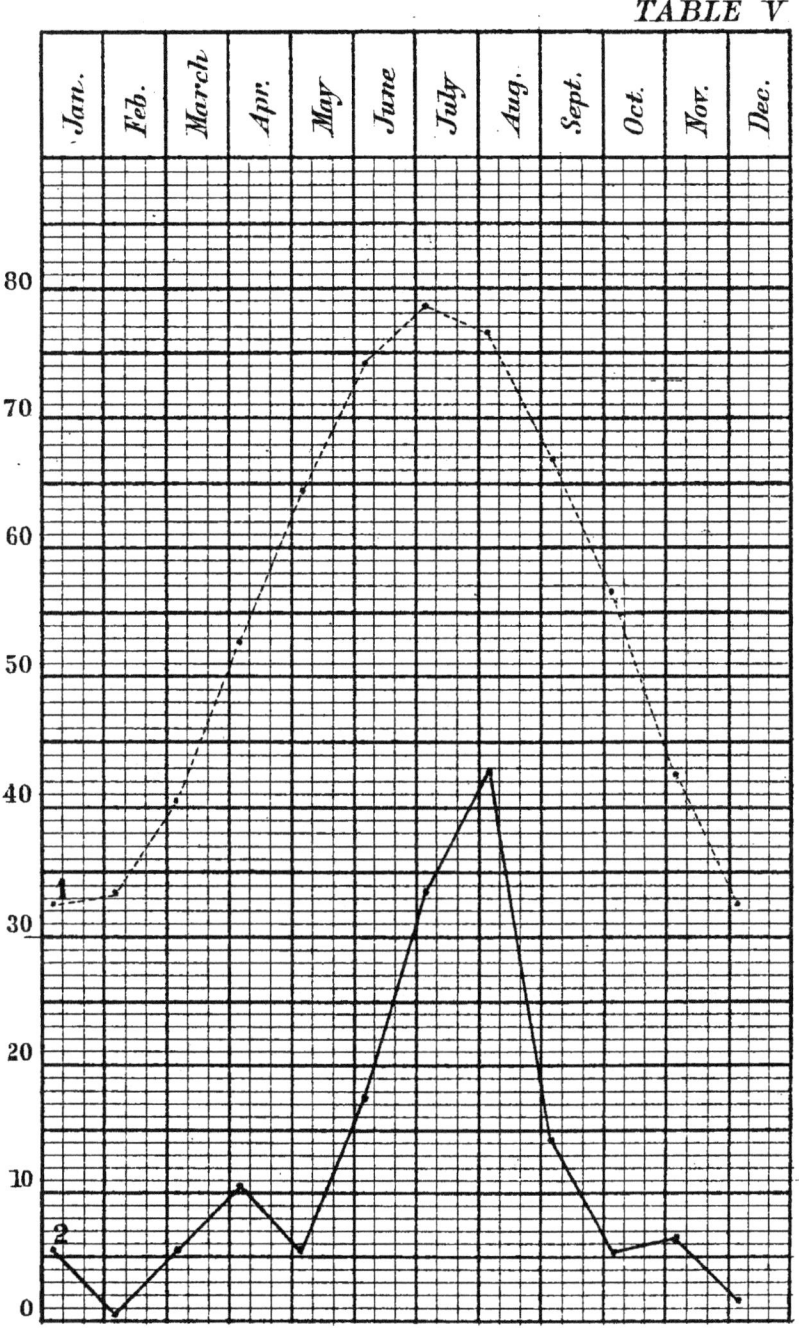

1 *Dotted line the temperature curve.*
2 *Black line Infantile palsy cases.*

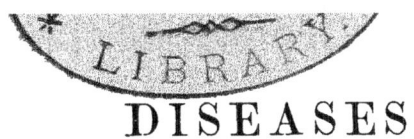

DISEASES

OF THE

NERVOUS SYSTEM,

ESPECIALLY IN WOMEN.

LECTURE I.

THE PARALYSES OF HYSTERIA.

THE case to which I drew your attention at my last clinic is here again, a girl, rather wanting in the signs of sexual ripeness, although sixteen years old. You will recall the fact that she lost the use of the right arm because of having been alarmed. The scare brought on what every woman knows as an attack of hysterics—our ancestors called it the vapors. The girl cried and laughed by turns, and then had a slight fit, on coming out of which she could no longer lift her right arm, or rather she could lift it but a few inches. On finding this to be the case, she grew much concerned, and by and by could not lift it at all, the idea that it could not be raised helping, as is apt to be the case, to make the trouble worse. There seems to have been no deceit, but perhaps the first feebleness may have been slight, and the power of her belief in her want of force great, and this is

2

rather the more likely since, as you saw, I raised the arm and said, "Now you can keep it up," which she did. You see that it seems again palsied. A new order restores it, and she lifts it without much effort, having won a belief in my being able to aid her. I send her away with a lightly uttered word or two as to the use of the hot iron, if she again loses power. The warning may answer or may not. We had a case very like this two years ago. I believe it got well.

We see here among the ill-fed, needy, and worried, a good many cases of hysterical loss of power, and I meet a yet larger number among women of the upper classes, where the disease is caused by unhappy love affairs, losses of money, and the daily fret and weari- someness of lives which, passing out of maidenhood, lack those distinct purposes and aims which, in the lives of men, are like the steadying influence of the fly-wheel in an engine.

It is my present wish to speak of some of the many kinds of hysterical paralysis, and to dwell far more freely on methods of treatment than upon minute details in the natural history of these disorders. I do this chiefly because as regards treatment I hold very positive opinions, and because these opinions have, I believe, been amply justified by happy re- sults, some of which are familiar enough to those who have followed my practice.

The group of instances of lessened power which I shall here discuss will include the usual forms of hys- teric paraplegia and hemiplegia, and that which I shall call double hemiplegia. I shall not attempt to cover the whole range of hystero-palsies, but seek chiefly so to define a certain number as to allow me to speak of their treatment. I shall also describe four forms of seeming loss of power, only one of which is essentially hysterical in nature, and not found elsewhere with the same features. I allude to hysterical motor ataxia.

The others are palsy from the rule of an idea, general paresis, and consciously mimicked palsy.

All three of these may be and are seen outside of hysteria, but they find in it a fertile soil, and are none the easier to treat when they are masking in this disguise.

One of the chief troubles in clearly knowing and in dealing with all of these forms of disease is due to the fact that in most cases, and to some extent, they may exist in union. The case of palsy may be partly real, partly pure weakness, partly loss of power from want of belief in being able to move; or conscious mimicry may be added to palsy or to the forbidding influence of a regnant idea, or to the true hysteric palsy may be joined ataxy of motion. For such vexing marriages of disorders, and for their offspring of doubt, we must be ready and watchful. They make the true limits of hysteric lack of power hard to define, hard to treat, full of surprises, and unfailing in interest and variety. Take this for an instance: You have a case of extreme hysteric paresis to treat. As a rule, it is readily cured. You predict a clear and happy future. As time wears on the mere weakness is gone, the limbs are plump again, the cheek red, and then you may find, if you have not been careful, as I have found, that hidden in the mere weakness there is a distinct amount of motor palsy—a mild, one-sided, loss of power—a true hysteric palsy, and not at all easy to cure. I shall pick for you, out of my note-books, cases of each of the forms of disease I have just spoken of, and shall try to make plain to you how I treat them. There were once no cases so much dreaded by me. There are now none to which I go with so much pleasure. I am sure that I treat them to-day with a success I could not once have gained, and I think that what success I have had has been due to more exact ideas as to what is needed, and that unflinching purpose and action which grow out of distinct views.

Let us take first a case of paraplegia—less common than hemiplegia and more difficult to relieve. The example I shall quote for you is the more interesting because of its having ended in death

Mrs. C., æt. 36, a strong woman, and in all ways well, lost by sudden death a child and her husband. Thus having cast on her the care of a large estate, loaded with many burdens, she began to show excess of anxiety as to her affairs, and from being sweet of temper became abrupt and full of unreasonable doubt as to her advisers. The worry brought with it speedy loss of blood globules, and as she was a woman who flowed very fully each month, all these causes together began to tell. This is the kind of thing we see much of in medicine. The books say this, that, or the other causes hysteria. In practice it is usual to find two or three causes—acting to assist one another. This woman was quite ready for an outbreak of some form of nerve trouble, when of a sudden she met the final blow in the form of a telegram. The news it bore was neither good nor ill, but by evil luck the writing looked like that of her dead husband, and she began to laugh with that strange want of appropriateness in emotional expression so common in the nervous. Awaking next day her legs seemed heavy, which caused her great alarm. At once, as she told me, the fear of palsy arose in her mind, and haunted her the more as, day by day, the feebleness grew worse. She was in Germany when taken ill, and seems to have been looked upon as suffering from an organic malady, for she was treated with nitrate of silver and the hot iron. Then as she failed to get relief anywhere, she was sent from one spa to another with a skill which as yet we are fortunately far from being able to reach.

St. Moritz, Schwalbach, Vichy, Louèche, and springs of lesser note, had each their turn, after the European fashion, until, in despair, she was carried back to America, where I saw her often and until the close of her life.

This was what I found: A woman of 35, height 5 feet 2 inches, weight 170 lbs., flabby, and thin blooded, with healthy heart, lungs, and kidneys. On the left side of the vagina was felt a tumor about the size of a walnut. It was very tender, and firm pressure on it gave rise to nausea and distress down the left leg. I had no doubt that this growth was a displaced ovary, but, despite this change of place, the left iliac fossa, both the skin and the parts reached by deeper pressure, was tender to touch. Was it ovarian tender-

2*

ness? Hardly, in this case. I have been told by Dr. Goodell that he has seen this same sensitiveness in other instances where the ovary had been displaced, and probably too much has been and is made of this symptom. The tenderness in Mrs. C.'s case was isolated, as is not unusual, and all about it up to the waist and down to the feet the body was without sense of touch or pain, or of heat and cold. In tracing this defect upwards it was found to cover the left breast, but this was so to-day, and then to-morrow it was less, the upper limit ranging from the navel to the left armpit.

Motor power was failing when I first saw her, but this had been the case before, and had been followed by a change for the better.

The plan pursued in treating the case was one to which I groped my way a few years ago. My patient was very thin blooded, and yet very fat. Such cases for some reason not clear to me are more hard to redden than are those of thin people in like states of blood. But if you can safely cause these persons to lose flesh, as they are helped to remake it, you may sometimes redden them with ease, and to raise the number of blood globules to the normal is usually to lift a woman above that low level of health, which is one, at least, of the factors of hysteria.

Mrs. C. was, when first seen by me, sitting up most of the day, and sewing, writing, and the like, when not too nervous. I put her in bed, and employing as a diet milk alone, mixed with a little rice-water or barley-water, I began to lessen the amount given, until, using less than a quart a day, her weight fell off at the rate of about a quarter to half a pound a day. When she showed signs of weakness I added beef soup to the diet for a day or two, and thus in one month brought down her weight some twenty-four pounds. This could not with safety be so quickly done unless the patient were kept inert and supine. Then the milk was by degrees increased. Raw beef and vegetables were added, malt extract was used before meals, a little red wine or champagne was allowed, and iron was given freely, the feeding being frequent. When I made the increase in diet I began to arouse sensation bv the use of the wire brush and induction currents.

Now in common palsies, or in those from nerve wounds, feeling is apt to come back first, motion last; but in hysteric palsies, as I think, the gain in active motion may go on, and even reach a useful amount while yet the lack of feeling rests as it was when the treatment began. Just this change took place in Mrs. C.: She grew brighter, and more happy, gained in color and flesh, and began to move her legs. In a month after she reached full diet she could walk with some trouble, and about this time the sense of touch showed signs of betterment, but the power to feel pain was unchanged, and, in fact, was never complete in the left leg.

Next began a plan of steady, urgent calls upon her for increase of the use of her limbs, so that before long she was able to walk out of doors. At this point I fear there was a mistake made in the treatment. Thinking the battle won I pushed her too hard, and one day after walking much further than usual she felt an excess of fatigue. Returning home she gave out of a sudden, and the morning after was again hardly able to stir either leg. I may pause here to repeat as to this matter a warning I have often given. It is to urge on you the utmost care as to allowing a hysterical patient on the way to health—I mean, of course, one who has lost power—to do more each day than fulfil the ordered task of that day. Most cases of hystero-palsies are easily tired, and it is almost sure to be the case that they cannot make a long effort without showing the effect in some way; moreover the mental results of extreme tire are to be feared, because any positive, real sensation is apt to become the peg, so to speak, on which the patient may hang the complement of a larger and less real sensation.

More slowly this time Mrs. C. got back some control over her movements, but at a certain point the gain ceased, and we made no further progress, nor did this surprise me. Hysterical paraplegia is, as I have said, more hard to cure than any other hysterical trouble except, perhaps, multiple contractures, and I felt that I had done well to win what I had won.

About six months later this lady died after a brief illness, which seemed to me more like a sudden and complete palsy of the pneumogastric nerves than anything else. No examination post mortem was allowed. I have known three deaths in hysteria; all were abrupt, and two were due to acute congestion of the kidneys.

Of that more common type, the palsies of one side of the body, you have seen a number. They are more frequent than paraplegias; less hard to cure, but quite lasting enough to make you cautious as to what you predict about their future. Where they occur in the feeble and thin-blooded, who have by degrees grown emotional, tearful, and weak of will, you may have more hope of helping them than if they are met with in robust people of non-emotional type, in whom the usual emotional elements which go to build up this temper of mind are wanting, or are small in amount. The former offer through the relief of their nutritive defects chances of obvious nature; the latter are apt to be bright or even able women, who enlist their mental forces in behalf of their symptoms, and treat the hated charge of being hysterical with utter scorn.[1]

I cannot leave this subject of hemipalsies of hysteria without a few words as to the ordinary type of this disorder. I shall therefore sketch for you somewhat briefly the chief symptoms of hemiplegia of hysterical origin.

This disease may come on slowly, and during the varied course of a case of hysteria, or it may arise abruptly, in an instant even, in women known or not suspected to be hysterical, owing to some profound emotion or to an accident, such as a fall or a wound. It is often of such insidious development that its presence, when mild, is a thing rather to be found by

---

[1] I ought, perhaps, to add that these women are usually mobile and excitable by nature, prone to laughter more than tears, so that it is hardly exact to say they are not emotional. Their form of too ready emotional disturbance lies merely in an unusual direction for the victims of hysteria.

looking for it than of such a nature as to be forced
upon the attention of the observer. It is excessively
rare to see it as complete as we see a hemiplegia of
organic origin. Nearly always, I might venture to
say always, it is associated with some loss or disturbance of sensation. More often this latter symptom
is the dominant one, and the lack of power merely
amounts to a paresis or incomplete palsy.

Unlike the hemipalsy of cerebral and organic cause,
hysterical half-palsies involve more or less all of one
side of the body, excepting the face; but in a few
rare cases the neck is distinctly affected, while usually when the case is incomplete, it is the leg which
suffers most, both as to sensation and motion.

Apart from the fact that the face escapes there are
other symptoms which differentiate these losses of
power from those which are due to clots or emboli,
and a knowledge of which enables us to diagnose the
case with sufficient ease, as arising from hysteria. As
to locality, in Briquet's cases there were 70 on the left
to 20 on the right; in my own note-books, I find the
proportion as 4 left to 1 right. The amount of loss
of power is often quite definite, but in other cases it
varies in degree within wider ranges than we see in
palsies of organic birth.

Sensation is disturbed, lessened, or lost either
throughout the one half of the body or in varying
amounts over this space, and in the face as a rule less
than elsewhere. In rare cases, the sensibility improves
very near the middle line of the body. In some instances no feeling exists; more often sense of touch and
power to localize sensations remains with profound

analgesia, and often also with lack of power to tell heat from cold. In bad cases the eye loses its keenness of perception, and the color sense is blunted while smell and taste alike suffer.

The ovarian region on one side is apt but not certain to be tender, either on the surface or upon deep pressure. Charcot and Dr. Buzzard both state that the patellar tendon reflex is exaggerated on the side of the palsy, and the latter that the ankle clonus may at times be met with. In the last three cases I have seen of hysterical hemipalsy the patellar tendon reflex was increased on the affected side. In two others it was notably lessened, as was the case in the girl present at my last clinic, where it was only possible to be sure that this symptom existed at all by grasping the muscles with one hand while the blow was struck. In another case the flexors responded and not the extensors ; and in yet another, with an exaggerated reflex, there was also a sharp contraction of the adductors on both sides.

These symptoms, with the history, should make the diagnosis an easy one, and I may add that while I see many mistakes made, owing to confounding hysteric paraplegias with those of organic cause, I rarely see such confusion as regards hysteric hemiplegia.

The following case, now in the Infirmary, may serve as a fair type of this form of paralysis. Miss L., a fine, large, ruddy woman of 26 years of age, owes her hemipalsy to the shock of a fall from affluence to the need to support herself by giving lessons in music. Then a succession of deaths fell upon her household, and at last one day, while teaching, she fell asleep, as

it were abruptly, at about 7 A. M. She was aroused
enough to be taken to bed, and there remained in
what seemed to be profound slumber, thirteen hours.
After this unusual trouble she grew more and more
hysterical, and at last came under my care. Her
organs are, in general, healthy; but she has this
curious peculiarity, of which she seems quite un-
aware. The pulse varies from 80 to 95, but the
respiration, without seeming to be hurried or distressed, is never less than 40, and is often 60 to the
minute.

She has considerable loss of power, with incomplete analgesia, defect of thermal sense, and preserva-
tion of touch. The face is scarcely affected at all,
and the senses of sight, smell, and taste are intact.
What is curious is, that there is no ovarian tenderness on either side, and that the analgesia varies
daily, almost hourly, as to extent, place, and amount.
A mustard plaster or blister, or, more remarkably, a
rhigolene freezing, will often restore feeling over a
large space for a few hours or for days; but inva-
riably the next menstrual flow undoes whatever
good may have been done. I tried the "metal cure"
in this, as I have tried it over and over in other and
worse cases; but although from it, or from glass,
cork, wood, or what not, I have obtained many times
a slight local change in feeling, I have never seen
this complete, and have never once witnessed the
phenomenon of transfer of the analgesia or anæsthesia
to the opposite side—a phenomenon which seems to
be undeniably frequent in the hands of as admirable
an observer as Charcot. I ought to add that my col-

league, Dr. Sinkler, has not been in this matter more fortunate than I, although he has, I believe, studied several cases from this point of view. The patient I have mentioned has many other hysterical troubles, and being quite rosy and stout, will be a difficult case to deal with. It is interesting to learn that until this girl came here neither she nor her medical attendants were aware that she had any loss of feeling.

The temperature of the left, the affected leg, is normal, or the same as the other, and pin-pricks fail to bleed at any part of the limb where there is lessened feeling. The tendon reflex of the patella is remarkably exaggerated on the palsied side, but there is no ankle clonus. Under use of good diet and tonics this girl is gaining color and weight, while by a succession of irritants, chiefly the wire-brush and induction currents, the sensation has been more and more successfully restored, so that the last menstrual flow has been less disastrous than usual.

I shall not trouble you further with details of this the most common type of hysteric hemiplegia, but pass on to one of the forms not well described as yet, and which I shall, in advance, venture to call double hemiplegia. This, as we shall presently see, is not merely another name for paraplegia.

Miss B., a sturdy, handsome girl, æt. 16 years, had a series of ills one on another from time to time. The first sign of trouble was twitches of the eyelids, and tears on reading; then there was a pause of two years. The next disturbance was a noisy and obstinate hiccup, during which both iliac fossæ became tender, and a single hypodermic use of morphia was

3

followed by convulsions.   Next came hysteric loss of
desire for food, nausea, pains in the left arm and leg,
and spasm of the vessels in the left leg, so that it became white and cold.   Up to this time she still walked
out; but in the summer of 1878 the use of galvanism
is said to have been followed by sick stomach and loss
of power to stand.   In the autumn she got rid of immense masses of hard feces, when all the symptoms
improved for a time.   The next winter was passed in
bed, vomiting a good deal; eating little; the bowels
very hard to move; the urine passed every hour.
About this time also she began to shun light, and
came at last to living, with covered eyes, in a dark-
ened room.   When I saw this young lady I was
struck with the thorough type of the emotional hysteric person she showed ; nor from the usual weak
will to the usual love of sympathy was there any tint
wanting to the picture.   I watched her for a few
days without ordering treatment until I learned all I
could of herself, her history, her home-life, her pur-
suits, her ambitions, and her mental powers.   Then
a talk with a watchful nurse helped me further, and
I saw clearly that I had to do not with a clever
woman who may be won over, and who is flattered
by the tribute paid to her mind when you insist that
to cure her she must be made to understand and
agree with you, but with a child who to be made well
had to be calmly and firmly ruled, and held day by
day to rigid account.   She was at once shut up, with
a good nurse, and kept at rest in bed, not being
allowed to use her hands even to feed herself.   As
she had been able to knit and sew, and be read to,

and to receive many visits, the sense of the irksomeness of the treatment soon made her eager to do anything I wished. Then began a system of bribes. She was told that if she could learn to bear the light she would be able to be read to, but that the nurse could not be allowed to strain her eyes. It would have been easy to open the windows and say you must bear the light, but if she herself gained this point of vantage, it would have the great value of being a self-conquest. In a few days I found the sunlight bright in her room. Then she was asked to overcome the habit of regurgitating her food. One or two scoldings, some show of disgust, and the promise that she should soon feed herself if she obeyed my wishes, helped us through with this. There were relapses; but as I found she hated milk I felt forced to put her back on the milk diet we began with whenever she threw up a meal, so that before long we heard no more of the vomiting; meanwhile the steady feeding and the use of massage, and local muscle treatment by electricity, began to show in a gain of flesh and color and firmness of muscle. She was now very weary of this unending quiet, and the time for education of the motor powers seemed to have come. Her loss of motion on the left side was very marked, and there was complete want of power to feel pain or to tell heat from cold; yet I could not make out any loss of vision or of color-sense. The touch was not perfect, but she knew fairly well where she was touched, although she could not be tickled.

As regards the pain sense there was one very curious point to which I have already alluded. As the needle

came within an inch or two of the middle line of the
body it was felt, and the better felt the nearer it came
to this line; nor do I recall having met with this
fact in any case of palsy from organic cause. The
right side of the body was palsied in a less degree,
and only as to motion, the leg far more than the
arm. The same was the case on the left side as
regards all the forms in which the functions were
deficient. Now as this case grew better the right
side became entirely well first, leaving the left hemiplegia as before, so that I have reason to speak of
the whole loss as being due to a double hemiplegia.
In other cases I have seen a general loss of sense and
motion, and observed entire relief on the right side,
leaving only a hemiplegia of the left.

My patient had some wasting of the left leg, and
less good electro-muscular reaction on the left, but
no pain on that side from any form of current. The
tendon reflex below the knee-pan was good on the
right; and also on the left: but what was new to me
the jerk was sometimes due to the extensors, and
sometimes due to the flexors, the extensors in the
latter case not seeming to move at all. Here was
another of the oddities of this most strange disorder.

As is usual she moved her limbs best while in bed,
and showed, when I came to let her sit up, or stand,
the loss of balancing power, which is seen in all
grave hysteric palsies, and is, indeed, almost a sure
sign of the parentage of the disease.

I have often asked you to note another point which
this case showed very well. You ask the patient to
raise the leg. It is lifted an inch; you insist on

effort, it is lifted higher; or if a great effort be made
the motion consists of a series of lifts and pauses.

The reliefs of distinct hystero-palsies are said to be
often abrupt. Under emotion or return of the menstrual flow, or on an order from some one, the patient
gets well. I must say that in hystero-hemiplegia
and paraplegia, with loss of feeling, I have not been
so happy as to see these delightful cures. In hysteria
with mere paresis, in the palsies from belief, or from
a ruling idea, I have seen such results many times.
Neither do I believe that all hysteria *is after a time*
within control of the sick person; nor that she can
in all instances run away in case of a fire, according
to a popular medical belief. In fact I have now in
my care a lady who was so tested by chance, and
who utterly failed to do more than fall down in her
effort to escape from a house on fire.

In fact profound emotions may work either way
for good or for ill, and no human sagacity will suffice to enable us to predict results. The evil is quite
as likely to be prominent as the good, and at all
events you may rest assured that emotions are somewhat unmanageable and unreliable as therapeutic
agents.

I have felt the need to say this, even if too briefly,
because I must add that the cures of these cases are
to be made by a slow, steady, hopeful training of the
will powers through every-day effort. which needs
some caution not to err in the way of excess. A
little nervousness is a bad sign, and it is well each
day to attempt a very little—no matter how little if
only we succeed, and can make the patient see it. I

shall in another place be more precise as to the means used. Enough to say of this case that it went on slowly gaining ground, and was under my care a year before the patient could walk well enough on crutches to go home with a cheerful future. It was not a brilliant case, and it taxed nurse and doctor to the uttermost—a case urged and scolded, and teased and bribed, and decoyed along the road to health; but this is what it means to treat hysteria. There is no short cut; no royal road

Let us take another case. It was as much like the last as it could well be. The patient, Miss C. P., æt. 18 years, the child of wealthy parents, came to me last year from Indiana. The motor losses were very remarkable, and, as in the last case, it was the left side which suffered most. She was unable to lift the left leg, or flex or extend the foot, so that below the knee there was motion in the toes alone. The left arm preserved all movements, but all alike were feeble. The right side was more symmetrically disordered, so that almost every muscle of the leg and arm was partially paralyzed. Sensation was lost for pain on the left side, save as to the belly and breast, where it seemed to be good, while in the face and neck it was lessened. Sense of temperature was more absolutely lost over the whole side than is common; and touch, not quite lost anywhere, was disturbed or lessened in irregular spaces. On the right side sense of pain was lessened in the arm and lost in the leg, while touch and the thermal sense were well preserved. There was one matter in which this case differed from the last one, and this changed my whole manner of dealing with the malady. My new patient was a clear-headed, well educated girl, who once had had a vigorous will. She was described to me as unselfish, thoughtful, and intelligent, and as a woman only brought down to a state of hysteria by long illness and the want of helpful advice at the right moment. She was emotional and ashamed of her tears, and honestly hated the whole matter of sickness. You will see such hysterical women. You will see others whose minds are like the back of a piece of needle-work with a baffling absence of pattern—women with a low, whining, bleating voice that is by itself a tell-tale of the kind of will-less ataxia which seems to cripple the mind no less than the body. These are the hard cases to relieve. But to return to my more favorable case. I tried to make her see how much the defects of body have to do with those of mind, and therefore the need to begin by building up the body anew. When, after a time, the limbs began to round, and color to come back to her pallid cheek, I set her to thinking how far the early troubles might have been within her control. I assured her that, although she could not now overcome at once the results due to habitual failure of self-control, repeated efforts would surely end in success. She was told that it was like the case of a bad temper, easy to hold in check at first, but if long unheld at last uncontrollable. It is not hard to open this point of view to a clever woman. You urge this idea from day to day; you ask her to try your way. She says she has done so, and then you point out that with ill health success was out of the question, while with rising health it might be easy. At last you get her to promise to fight every desire to cry, or twitch, or grow excited.

Above all, you teach her the priceless lesson for a woman of the value of moods, of the ease with which she can get herself into a state of dangerous tension, of the necessity of learning, not how to bear a thing, but how to approach the idea of bearing it in a state of calm. It is a long sermon, but I can only give these few pregnant texts. It is always apt to win with a woman of intelligence, and the fools are to be dealt with by other moral drugs than these, or the honest pill must be gilded with timely flattery or such better motives as may help it to find the woman's conscience, if that is to be stirred at all.

By and by, as one symptom after another gave way before her efforts, she became more and more sure that I must be right as to all; and I have seen few cases gain ground with equal speed. Nevertheless a whole year was needed to make her well able to take up afresh her full round of social and household duties. In fact, even with the best of self-help from the patient, the cure of any one of these cases is a long and arduous course of education.

Before leaving the subject of hysteric palsies I would say a few words as to the electric reactions. In most cases, and early in nearly all, the muscle reactions are normal; but after a time, and in most old cases, these are less good than in health; nor do limbs long palsied fail to shrink somewhat, while marked wasting is rare. When there is loss of motion and of feeling, Duchenne's axiom is correct; that is, we have then normal electric reaction of muscles and absence of all sensation of pain from the most severe currents. In some early cases I have seen a state of things not elsewhere spoken of. I saw it last week in a chronic case of horrible rhythmic spasms of the arms, with palsy of sense and motion in the legs. Dr. Yarrow, the attending physician, studied with me the electric state, which was curious. When with slow or rapid breaking of circuit (induced currents) we tested the leg muscles, the poles, even with currents unbearable by us, caused no motion until they had been steadily applied for from two to three minutes over any one muscle; but the reaction of nerve and muscle, one pole on each, was somewhat more rapid, although still very slow. What we saw was in reality but an exaggeration of the delay in arousing muscles which we see in health and in other forms of disease than hysteria.

LECTURE II.

HYSTERICAL MOTOR ATAXIA HYSTERICAL PARESIS.

THE form of disorder to which I shall first direct your attention in connection with the false palsies of hysteria is the motor ataxia of this disease. It is necessary here to be extremely precise, because, as you will see if you read Briquet's admirable study of hysteria, he also describes a form of hysterical motor ataxia.

Ataxia, as you well know, means merely disorder or irregularity, and when therefore we speak of loco-motor ataxia we mean only disordered movement, and not of necessity enfeebled movement. The cause of the disorder or incoördination thus introduced into motor functions may vary.

In hysteria, so far as I know, there are two forms of motor ataxia independent of those associated with vertigo. That described by Briquet and Laségue seems to depend upon a loss of sensation in both skin and muscles. In Laségue's case the girl was only able, the eyes being closed, to move the limbs which were still sensible, but was totally unable to move the anæsthetized parts or to know where they were when moved by another person. While seeing, she could walk readily and even without looking at her feet.[1] In other and similar cases there is merely a lack of coördination in complex motor acts.

There is, however, another and a very interesting form of hysterical motor ataxia which is, I fancy, rather rare in its most perfect type, and which may without due care be taken, as Duchenne's disease was long taken, for some kind of paralysis.

The trouble I am about to speak of I find to be in some of its degrees very common in hysteria—to co-exist with many hysteric palsies or paretic states, and sometimes, though rarely, to be the prominent malady, with almost no loss of voluntary power.

The hysterical ataxic patient of this class, and I shall consider first the nearly pure case, has full feeling, or may have it, and is quite well able to use the limbs more or less freely while lying down. When she begins to sit up or kneel or stand, the lack of coördinate muscular movements becomes at once visible.

Instantly the patient begins to fall to one side, a voluntary effort to redress the disturbed balance results in a partial fall to the other side or back or forward, as may chance. The patient *seems* to be unable to judge of the extent to which the balance is lost, and also to determine or evolve the amount of power needed to overcome the defect. The abruptness of these efforts at redressing the loss of equilibrium

---

[1] There may be in this something of habit. In the few cases of Duchenne's disease which I have seen in women I have been struck with the way in which, as their garments habitually hide the feet, they managed to dispense with the guiding sight of these parts.

appears to show an absence or defect of the usual antagonistic activity of opponent muscles. I am inclined to suggest as a reasonable theory that perhaps a large share of this difficulty may be due to a slowness in volitional acts by reason of which the mandate reaches the muscle too late to be of ready service. This is by no means unlikely, for in some hystero-palsies I have measured and proved the retardation of nerve conduction. Slowness in learning the need to move a muscle and slowness in moving it would give rise to just such incoördinate action as these cases exhibit. The lack of orderly movement is chiefly in the neck and trunk, and is made worse, like all disorder of motion, by excluding the guiding influence of vision.

This very interesting form of incoördination in muscular acts is limited for the most part to the more complex movements. It is seen little or least in single limb motions, better in sitting or kneeling, better still in standing, and best of all in walking. It is not due to weakness because it exists in cases strong enough to sit, stand, and walk firmly, if only power were needed to the efficient accomplishment of these acts. Also, while you may find it with general or local lack of surface feeling, it is not due to this, because anæsthesia of the skin is, in the hysterical at least, incompetent to cause ataxia of motion. In the confusion and odd grouping of symptoms in hysteria, the trouble I have described is apt to be overlooked or attributed to coincident conditions. It is, therefore, fortunate to find now and then cases in which this form of motor disorder occurs almost alone, so that we have a chance of studying it without being embarrassed by other symptoms.

I believe that this ataxic state is common in grave hysteria, and is to be found often enough in milder cases. I think also that some of the cases which are attributed too promptly to muscular anæsthesia will be found to be free from that defect, and to be due to other causes than those to which Briquet has attributed them. Perhaps it may be that conscience of locality will prove a differentiating test, since it is said to be lost in the hysterical ataxia of Briquet, and is certainly not lost in the form I have here delineated.

I do not think one could readily confound this ataxia of movement with anything else unless it be with one of the rarest of the forms of hysterical spasm. The following case is an apt illustration of this latter disease which might perhaps be well described as alternating spasms, the action of the flexors calling the extensors instantly into movement, and these in turn summoning the flexors into like activity. These semi-spasmodic motions were the more curious in the last case I saw because of the general and profound paresis which made every volitional effort excessively difficult. I may add that there was also a contraction of the right leg and a left hemi-anæsthesia with conscience of place.

The patient, when seated and held up, or even when the head alone was unsustained, showed the following symptoms: The head or body was pulled to one side. At the limit of this motion, or before that was reached, it was violently jerked over by the

opponent muscles, as if their stretching were the sig-
nal for an explosive act of power. At once or in a
moment the other muscles acted in like fashion, and
so the head or trunk was thrown about in a strange
and disorderly manner so long as the patient remained
upright. The same type of movement extended to
the legs and arms. These acts were certainly of
volitional birth, but they were, so to speak, convulsive renderings of natural acts, and were sometimes
very violent.

I may add that, notwithstanding the complexity of
symptoms, with such a loss of memory as necessitated
an entire re-education, this girl became entirely well.

In place of giving you types of motor ataxia with
palsy I shall prefer to choose one now in my care, and
which has the least share of palsy for the largest
share of incoördination of the muscles.

Miss B., æt. 20, Kentucky, of healthy, living
parents, in August, 1876, while going home from the
Centennial Exhibition, caught a slight cold, out of
which came complete loss of voice for seventeen
months. In its return it came and went abruptly,
and was well to-day and gone to-morrow. In September, 1871, at the Hot Springs, Arkansas, after a
good deal of worry, she is said to have had headache and dizziness, after which of a sudden she lost
speech, and became unconscious, with her jaws firmly
locked. The legs and arms were seized with spasms,
and when they became better had nearly lost touch-
sense, and did not feel pin pricks. This attack ended
in weakness and fever, with cold feet and loss of power
to swallow even saliva. After three weeks she re-

gained speech, and then again relapsed. She was said to have had a typhoid fever, which does not seem likely.

About the fifth week she was found to have lost power in the legs. The loss is described as having been nearly entire, but by March, 1879, she had regained a good deal of motion. Since then she has been at a standstill.

In October I saw Miss B. in bed, a dark-skinned, rosy-looking girl, without the least turn to tears or undue emotion. I should only have said that her manner was quick and excitable. She certainly had none of the usual furtive look, and small deceitfulnesses of some hysterical girls. Neither was there any loss of tendon (patellar) reflex, and the senses of pain, of touch, and of heat were perfect.

While in bed Miss B. moved all her limbs somewhat slowly, but with a great deal of power; the lift of the leg was done in jerks, as by distinct orders of will, but she showed none of the tremor and twitching of face and tearful look so common in hysteric girls called on for an unusual effort. When held up on her knees, she swayed to and fro, always falling if not assisted. When somewhat later she could stand up, the motor disorder showed still better. From head to foot every muscle used to preserve the upright posture gave way momently, and was braced again by distinct acts of will. The rocking motion so caused was curious to see. A slight push was sure to upset her, as if she was unable to provide in time enough of power to resist the shock and restore the disturbed balance. If I warned her of the coming shock, she did far better. The touch of a hand greatly aided her, and the closing of her eyes made things worse. Nor did Miss B., when standing, appear to have the least idea of her balance being in danger until the sway of her figure became extreme, when she caught herself up, and with an effort regained her erect position only to fall to the other side. There seemed to be a lack of appreciation of the failing balance, and a slowness in redressing it when lost or in peril. When added to this we have complete loss of feeling, when skin, bone, joint, and muscle share alike in this respect, we have, of course, a still more complete and a different form of want of power to preserve the upright posture, but this is the character of the trouble spoken of by Briquet and others, and I wished to make it clear that there were causes of motor ataxy which did not of need involve any lack of tactile sense.

In Miss B.'s case little was needed beyond training the weak and inapt muscles, because she ate and digested well, slept soundly, and was free from pain.

My first step was to point out to her that, after she had made an effort which seemed extreme, another forth-putting of will would add to the previous result. This seems a simple thing to make clear; but, if you can convince your patient of the fact, it is of great service, because then you go on to point out further that, perhaps, by a series of trained and aided efforts, there may be won, bit by bit, a full power of motion. To lodge this idea in a woman's mind is at once to widen the horizon of hope. How much you gain by it depends a little on whether your patient is clever and wants to get well, or is silly and prefers the role of hysteria; but, after all, the whole mode of treatment rests on a study of character, or of character and hysteria, and a moral diagnosis is the first step to take.

With Miss B., at a standstill for months—bright clever, longing for active life—the idea was as a wholesome ferment. The nurse now began to train her while in bed to move the legs, one at a time, very slowly, but in larger and larger movements, with intervals between of a minute or more.

An order is given to lift the leg; if it be too weak, a finger beneath the ankle aids it, but no attempt must be let to fail utterly; as she gets on, the orders are to be obeyed more quickly. It is easy to sketch out for one's self what such a system should be in its details. After it has gone far enough, the patient is seated in bed with some support to her spine, and is trained to move the head freely. When, in Miss B.'s case, she was put on the edge of the bed seated, the motor ataxia began to show, so that it took some time to overcome this trouble. The next step used with me to be a lesson in walking, but of late I find it better to teach the girl to creep, which is an easy and natural mode of training for the walk. The patient has pads tied over her knees, and, lying flat on her face on the floor, without skirts, has around her a folded sheet. At an order, she tries to rise, helped by the lift of the sheet-belt held by the nurse. When she is able to do this, and can gather her legs and arms so as to make herself a quadruped, she is taught to balance herself, every effort being assisted,

when needing help, by the nurse standing above her.
The progress to creeping is easy; then comes the
lesson of kneeling and pushing a chair; and last that
of standing in a corner or by a chair. You see that,
following nature's lessons with docile mind, we have
treated the woman as nature treats an infant. For
aid in walking we have three devices: the expensive
wheel crutch, which can be easily imitated by a clever
carpenter, being merely a framework with rollers so
arranged that it includes crutch supports. Next, if
need be, I use a device which may be common, for
all I know, but which I have not seen elsewhere. It
is a pair of crutches with a stout half-hoop of metal
between and in front of the two. This gives a solid
support, and, in ataxic cases, is very useful as giving
a sense of security, and therefore of confidence.
This crutch-frame is soon replaced by a pair of supports, the bases of which are about seven or eight
inches long and two broad. They may be made like
the lower half of a crutch, or have two columns of
a support set in the base, or may be a single cane with
broad base; the top in any case should have a double
curve so as to lie easily in the line of the natural slope
of the palm when resting on such a support. A rubber
footing gives a little elasticity and a good hold on
any form of flooring. With such a broad base of
support, it is quite pleasant to find how soon the
patient learns with its aid to balance herself. A
third form of support which I devised two or three
years ago is of use in hysteric or in any form of
hemiplegia. If the left arm be too feeble to aid the
left leg by grasping a crutch, I resort to the following

arrangement. On the lame side a crutch, having above an unusually deep hollow to receive the armpit, is fastened to the arm by two straps or by a glove riveted to the hand-piece of the crutch, so as that the hand once slipped into it is pretty firmly held. From the crutch a double metal bar curves forward and towards the sound side, and ends in a handle which is grasped by the sound hand and carried forward by it. I have found these supports most useful in many forms of weakness. In making them or having them made, pray remember that they should be made light; most crutches are too heavy.

With regard to Miss B., I may add that she got well in two months so as to walk unhelped anywhere, and that she is now free from pain and nervousness.

Before leaving the subject of hysteric motor ataxy, I wish to add yet a single illustrative case in order to show that ataxy, connected with hemiplegia, may affect a single limb. Such cases approach in character the choreoid troubles which accompany or follow certain cases of hemiplegia from organic dis-ease of the brain, and afford yet another of the shadowy resemblances which link the various forms of hysterical disorders to their analogues of more definite parentage. Miss C., æt. 30, grew up in luxury and ease, subject to what she somewhat indefinitely described as spells of prostration with nervousness. At the age of twenty a sudden death in her family caused a sharp convulsive attack, followed by a brief period of insanity, lasting in all three weeks. Three years later her family fell into almost absolute want, and she began to work hard in the effort at self support, and then gradually failed in health, suffering at intervals from a variety of hysterical symptoms. These resulted abruptly in incomplete left hemi-anæsthesia, with great loss of power in the leg and lessened power in the hand and arm.

With this report of her case she came to me some months ago. Except a very slight retro-flexion, there was no uterine trouble. Neither ovary was sensitive, but the spine in all its length, and the left side of the chest and the upper part of the belly were very tender—more to touch than deep pressure. All other organs were healthy.

The hemi-anæsthesia as to touch and pain was notable in the parts below the waist, and was incomplete in irregular areas, which shifted daily. Pin pricks did not bleed in the leg.

The hand and arm had good sense of touch everywhere, but lessened pain sense chiefly on the radial aspect of the arm. The leg was almost motionless. The arm and hand could be used with nearly natural force, but were stricken with remarkable ataxy of movement without the least sign of spasm. The utmost concentration of will failed to direct the hand so as to enable it to grasp or manipulate an object once held. The limb would waver to and fro, and at last descend on the object with an effort which usually carried the hand far to left or right. A certain abrupt jerkiness characterized every motion, and the failure of directive power was singularly illustrated at the piano, where the one incoördinate member contrasted with the unusually skilful touch of the other. As so often happens in the post-paralytic chorea of cerebral lesions, the palsy was inversely as the ataxic difficulty, and consisted rather in lack of persistent energy than in want of initiatory power.

By slow degrees this ataxv of movement passed away, and what was most curious it lessened with the increase in want of power, while this also has in turn disappeared, leaving as yet some dysæsthesia, but no notable want of strength.

There yet remains to us hysteric paresis. Among the many disorders which hysteria affords, certain ones come clearly out at times from the tangle of named or nameless symptoms, and enable us to speak of them under some distinct name. It is a comfort, amidst so much that is confusing, to find these groupings of symptoms, and, in diseases of vague boundaries like neurasthenia and hysteria, a good deal of this useful sort of secondary classification is possible.

The history of hysteria is sometimes one of years, and in certain cases, either at the outset or after more or less of the strange drama of this disease has been played, the patient falls into a state of inertness of mind and body, which I am forced for lack of a better name to call hysteric paresis.

You might, I presume, feel free to give to these cases another label than the one I have given. They are, however, over and above all else paresis—pure intense feebleness; but it is paresis in hysterical women, and if you forget this fact, when it exists, you may be sure that you will have but little success in the treatment.

This disorder may be seen in union with other signs which are more or less clearly hysterical; but sometimes we find it almost pure from these disguises, as in the case of Miss L., from New Jersey, now in the Infirmary. A person of languid nature, not strong in mind or body, she began some years ago to be emotional, to have loss of appetite, weakness, tender spine, vertex headaches, and abdominal tenderness and rare convulsions. By and by she took to bed, and with more and more complaint of her back, and soon of soreness everywhere, ate less and less, gave no care to her bowels, and at last became feeble, sallow, wasted to the limit of wasting, and content to lie still most of the time, using mind and body as little as she could. From this state I rescued her and made her well, and now she is here again far worse than ever, unable to lift a limb or to turn over. She is twenty-two years old, and has not menstruated in six months. She is five feet five inches, and may weigh about eighty-eight pounds. Her skin is rough, dry, unpliant, yellowish, and seems to be firmly glued to the bones and muscles beneath it. Her morning temperature does not exceed 97.5° F.; her heart beats 90 to 120, and is quick and feeble. The other organs seem healthy, and the secretions normal. She cries at times, but not much. Her face, marked with acne, is set, inert, wooden, as if she could not smile. The lids droop, the mouth hangs a little open, the voice is so feeble that it is hard to know what she says. The spine is very tender, and to touch it causes a gush of tears; but the left iliac fossa and the chest muscles are also tender, and compression of any of these hyperæsthetic spaces causes nausea and vertigo. Her dislike to make any effort was great, but it was clear that no motion was lost, although all were wonder-fully feeble. There was not during movement the jerky action of hystero-palsies, but an extreme and evident difficulty in motion, and a sudden failure to prolong it.

I was very much struck in this case with the ease with which these patients become feverish. The least over-exertion was competent to cause a distinct rise in temperature and pulse; but, for some reason not yet clear to me, these changes required some hours to produce them.

All the battery of toning influences was turned on this woman, and she is now gaining ground apace. She is fed often and in small amount, had for a time rectal feeding also—and the mechanical tonics, mas-sage, and electricity. As usual in all such cases, we wait until the flesh is coming back, the color bright-ens, and the muscles grow firmer under our mechani-cal stimulations before we call upon her to exert her-self. Then, in this order, with passive motion—motion aided by a nurse, motion resisted by a nurse, active motion, unhelped—we shall train her back to a state of health. We shall cure her surely, but whether or not she will remain well I cannot say. It will depend on what kind of influences surround her, on what she is when well.

I have given here a short sketch of a state of paresis, in which with some anæmia or without a very marked condition of lack of blood all the func-tions are enfeebled, and this is most notable in those which involve muscular exertion of any kind. If there be also any pain, such as that of spinal irritation

made worse by motion, the patient is even more apt
to be sluggish, and is not slow to avail herself of this
and of every excuse to keep as quiet as possible.
The real and singular want of power, as measured by
the dynamometer, the difficulty in beginning as well
as in continuing a motion, seems to set this apart
from cases of mere neurasthenia, while the general
wasting and appearance of mal-nutrition serve yet
more deeply to mark the distinction. The disorder
I have described so briefly is one of those which adds
many recruits to that large class which some one has
called "bed cases," and which are above all things
distinguished by their desire to remain at rest.

I shall elsewhere give in sufficient detail what I
over and over allude to in these lectures—my views as
to how best to treat those difficult combinations of
hysteria with defective nutrition which are often too
much for the best of us, and to those pages, and to what
I have written previously in other places, I must now
refer you. I have some belief in the occasional value
of induction-currents in hystero-palsies, but, as to the
direct good to be had out of the drugs on which men
once relied in the treatment of this disease, I have
said nothing, because, except to condemn, I had
nothing to say, and because I believe that the numberless remedies for hysteria to be found in the books
will be swept by another generation into the limbo
provided for drugs with decayed reputations; but in
thus expressing myself I do not mean to say that no
drugs have an indirect value. What you have to do
is to rectify with care positive uterine troubles, to
treat defects of nutrition, to relieve the anæmia so

apt to exist in hysteria, to see that every function is well cared for, and last, not least, to learn what need there is to alter the moral surroundings of your patient, and then with kind and patient care, and an unbending will, to bring about the changes she may seem to require.

5

LECTURE III.

MIMICRY OF DISEASE.

YOU will recall the fact that the case I show you
to-day is one of three which have presented themselves at this clinic within one week. Each of these
by chance illustrates a different form of disorder, and
each of the three is a distinct example of one of the
various groups of causes which evolve a simulation
of disease. The literature of this subject is widely
scattered, and consists chiefly of isolated cases to be
found in the journals. The best essays on the surgical aspect of simulated disorders are the admirable
lectures of Paget, Skey's little volume, and an able
paper by Dr. Schaffer, of New York, on hysterical
disease of joints. Except Russell Reynolds's paper on
diseases due to fixed ideas or emotions, I know of no
medical essay of much merit on this subject. It is
to be desired that the whole subject should be handled
afresh by some competent physician. It would be
easy for me to make up for you an interesting history
of these troubles from the experience of others, but
I think that I shall be more pleasantly instructive if
I deal only, or most largely, with cases coming within
the range of my own knowledge, and especially if I
make use of some of the curious self-analyses which
patients who have recovered have placed at my dis-

posal. Both for what they betray and what they conceal these histories are valuable, and especially so when they come from women of educated intelligence.

The elements out of which these disorders arise are deeply human, and exist in all of us in varying amount, while many of the determining and conditioning factors come from accidental, or, at least, external agencies. As a rule, the means at work to produce mimicked disease are in the books made to seem too simple.

I have not time to do here as I might wish, and to go into the full psychology of this subject, and must content myself, therefore, with an outline which shall mark out for you the chief causes which supply the foundations for simulated diseases, and those which build on this, and those which strengthen and guard the morbid structure.

First of all comes the hysterical state, fertile parent of evil. However produced, it is a fruitful source of mimicry of disease, in its every form, from the mildest of dreamed pains up to the most complete and carefully devised frauds. Its sensitiveness and mobility, its timidity and emotionalness, its greed of attention, of sympathy, and of power in all shapes supply both motive and help, so that while we must be careful not to see mimicry in every hysteric symptom, we must, in people of this temperament, be more than usually watchful for this form of trouble, and at least reasonably suspicious of every peculiar or unusual phenomenon.

What it is convenient to call the nervous temperament, or that state which may be acquired, and which

I like to describe as general nervousness, is a fertile
field for simulated maladies, because in it, as in hysteria, the qualities which we all possess are apt to take
on a morbid development, and to get out of the limits
of rational control.

Of the individual share taken by each of these
causes I shall by and by speak. Before, however, I
pass on to lesser premises, I would like to digress in
order to say a few words in explanation of what I
mean by general nervousness. You will find this
term used over and over in these lectures, and also in
the annual statement of diseases treated at the Infirmary for diseases of the nervous system. I used
to try to classify these cases under other heads, but
came at last to see that there is a state which is best
labelled thus, and that after eliminating all the cases
which can be otherwise classed, a small residuum is
left to which no other name applies. Some of them
are more or less neurasthenic people, easily tired in
brain or body; but others without this, or with this
peculiarity but slightly developed, are merely tremu-
lous nervous folks, easily agitated, over-sensitive,
emotional, and timid. This state falls on man or
woman or child, and is not hysteria. It is with some
people a morbid birth-gift, with some an inheritance,
and in its worst shapes it is made or acquired by mis-
use of alcohol or tobacco, or tea or coffee. Naturally
you may think that such a state must be slowly created, and usually it is; but also it is true that a very
permanent state of general nervousness may be
evolved by the accident of a moment, when precedent conditions favor it. In a lecture on general

nervousness in the male, I mentioned examples of this kind, and last week we saw at my clinic a case in which a moment of intense terror, owing to the fall of a house wall, caused in a healthy girl a state of general nervousness, alike serious and lasting. However acquired, the condition I have outlined highly favors the mimicry of disease.

Another good growing ground for simulation is in a mere lowering of the general tone of health from anæmia, or any cause whatsoever. You know that out of failing health comes, often enough, nervousness or hysteria, but even when these states do not arise, mere lowering of the standard helps, in many susceptible people, to awaken doubts, suspicions, and terrors, which need little hint or help from without to enable the victim to construct a morbid edifice of non-existent disease.

If, then, you should ask me whether for the creation of mimicked disorders we need the aid of lowered health, of hysteria, or of general nervousness, I should answer that while such states are usually the responsible parents, a small proportion of examples arise in persons who being in absolute health owe the troubles in question to their possessing some natural or inherited combination of physical peculiarities, which becomes a competent mischief maker when aided by external accident. The people who, from any cause, simulate disease are, I think, apt to be naturally distinguished by certain peculiarities. They are generally over-sensitive, pain hurts them more than others, and is a more important matter in life. Perhaps they really feel pain more, and, at all events, they complain of it more. As a rule, they are timid, fearful, and watchful, nursing for evil, any chance word incautiously dropped, and, therefore, prone to dwell on physicians' opinions, to deduce exaggerated possibilities of trouble, and in obedience to the least prediction of ill to consent or hasten to take extreme precautions.

Then, again, you are aware that every one has some capacity for mentally influencing or disturbing functions of the body which usually are not under the control of volition. A few well people have this in a marked manner, and in some hysteric or nervous states this power becomes enormously increased and widened in range. I do not mean that these people acquire the power to will intestinal trouble, for instance, but that they certainly may gain ability to somehow disturb the bowel functions by thinking of them. There are many stories in regard to this; but let the average man endeavor by any mental process to cause diarrhœa, and he will, I think, find it no easy task. It seems incredible that a woman can learn to vomit at will; but this is common; and, also, happily she can be taught to suppress this vomiting by volitional effort when the will is aided by a potent motive.

Books like Dr. Tuke's are full of stories illustrative of such facts, and I myself have seen a large number. It is clear, then, that we can sometimes acquire such control over functions supposed to be outside of volitional rule, and that this is made easier in certain temperaments and in states of hysteria, feebleness, or nervousness.

The disturbances thus brought about lie usually in

the heart or vessels, or in the gastro-intestinal track, and are caused or aided by expectant attention or dread, or by morbid watchfulness with a knowledge of symptoms.

It has been said by Hunter, as quoted by Tuke, that, if a number of men surrounding a table on which they have placed each a hand will fix their attention on the member, some of them at least will soon feel in the part a peculiar sensation. I have tried this in vain, and I have also tried without result to cause my heart to beat quicker by merely attending to its action, yet I am myself of a rather nervous temperament. It is curious to find John Hunter avowing the ease with which he could in this manner create symptoms, and then to find Sir James Paget declaring himself utterly unable to produce mimicry of disease by any amount of attentive effort. The difference among healthy men in this respect must, however, be immense. Of this I had once a curious illustration. When a very young man, five of us made a series of what are called by the homœopathists provings of certain medicines, each man being ignorant of the drug taken; three of the five had a great variety of symptoms, but the other two had none. It is well to add that the symptoms corresponded neither among the observers nor to those set down in the homœopathic manuals. My friend, Professor Tyson, will recall an amusing example of the effects of expectation in a patient of ours. The first day he saw her, in order to use electricity, she chanced to have at the time, as she always had under excitement, a loose stool. This took place also at his next visit; and thereafter he never made a call at a set time without causing sharp purgation. When he came unlooked for, then the whole trouble left her. It brought to my mind the case of a well-known English physiologist, who happened to have diarrhœa when about to give his first lecture. The embarrassment and annoyance were great, and so impressed him that for a year he never lectured without having just beforehand a loose stool. The sufferer chanced to relate these facts to a well-known physician, then a very young man; being himself also a biologist, he unluckily felt interest enough in this matter to recall it when soon after about to appear for the first time before an audience. The excitement attendant on a novel situation, with a knowledge of how it had affected another, caused it to have a like effect on him, and for a long time he was always thus annoyed when about to lecture.

I have given these as illustrations of increase of action under mental disturbances and expectation or dread. They could readily be multiplied. In the two cases named, anxiety caused the repetition of a flow which was at first accidental, or, at all events, not born of emotion alone. In like fashion arise and continue certain of the forms of cardiac and vasal nervous disturbances. First there is some sudden and unusual influence disturbing the circulation, then, upon occurrence of lesser but like causes, a similar trouble arises, until a morbid habit is fully formed.

There exists in all of us, feebler in age and more potent in childhood, a tendency to automatic and unconscious imitation which is the parent of a good deal of the mimicry of disease. It may exist in simple forms, or be accented by love, anxiety, fear, or even disgust.

I have said it was potent in the young, and it is in them responsible for a good many of the peculiarities and resemblances usually set down to inheritance; but it is also to be seen at times in their elders. Some months ago I was showing to a physician a very singular case of unilateral grimace. As I turned from my patient, I noticed that the doctor was repeating with his own features the morbid action before him. I said, "Do you know that you were imitating this lad's grimace?" "I know now," he said, "but I must have done it without conscious imitation." Perhaps no better or more illustrative example of the natural tendency could be given. This was pure automatic imitation.

The tendency to cough, when forced for a long time to listen to a cough, is an instance where tendency to imitation is made powerful by sympathy or affection. It may account for some at least of the false whooping-coughs we meet with.

A far more amusing example is one which I have seen several times, but which seems to have escaped mention in print. It is the occurrence of vomiting in the husband of a pregnant woman. The story of one of these unlucky sympathizers is worth telling :—

He was rather noted as an unfaithful mate and a man of altogether loose ways. After five years of marriage, his wife becoming pregnant—an event much desired—he seemed to reform, and was very much in her society. Her vomiting, which was extremely severe, at last affected him, every day or two, to his utter disgust. Her second pregnancy gave rise to a return of his malady. I believe that she ceased to be sick with her third child—certainly with her fourth—but, so soon as on each occasion he became aware of her state, his vomiting came on, and lasted for a month or two; indeed, I think, in one case much longer.

The character of his disorder at length became known to his friends, and he was so mercilessly chaffed that it was at last almost dangerous to mention the matter. I have seen other cases—his was the worst—but I was told of one in New York last week, and the victim was a physician.

I may have overlooked something in my search through the books for mention of these curious facts. Prof. Goodell reminds me of what Francis Bacon says (Cent. x. Para. 986): "There is an opinion abroad—whether idle or no I cannot say—that loving and kind husbands have a sense of their wives breeding child, by some accident in their own bodies." Did he mean vomiting, or some more mysterious diagnostic warning? In the *Lancet* there is brief mention incidentally of a husband as having been sick at stomach during his wife's pregnancy.

There could be no better examples than these somewhat ludicrous instances of the influence of automatic imitative tendencies. In the case just mentioned, the habit became so strong that emesis was re-excited by a mere knowledge of the fact that there existed in the woman the state out of which previously had grown the original trouble

Instances of graver disease evoked in like fashion have been given by Reynolds and Anstie, and always it is found that fear, or the sight or the remembrance of suffering in others, has been an efficient means of aiding the imitative tendency. In this manner troublesome paresis, simulative of palsy seen in a relative, has been produced. The condition thus acquired is not a true palsy, and does not give us the full roll of symptoms seen in the real case; but it is something more than a mere voluntary imitation, because there is often a distinct incapacity for movement. The difficulty as to the amount of true pain felt in such of these cases as mimic that symptom, I shall more than once have occasion to speak of; and it follows us everywhere in our efforts to fairly appreciate the extent of nerve irritation. It must bear to true pain perhaps some such mysterious relation as the paresis of these cases bears to true paralysis.

I saw last winter a young lady of highly nervous and timorous organization, who was long under my care, and at length fully recovered. While in bed an indiscreet attendant told her of the horrible agony she had witnessed in a case of facial neuralgia, which began daily about 11 A. M. A day or two later my patient began to have pain in the same locality and at the same hour every morning. She was one of those women in whom you could cause pain anywhere by pressure on the spine, and a few suggestive and directing remarks; and no more was needed than the frequent mention of the torment of another, and the remembrance that she herself had already had what was called ovarian neuralgia. For some days she really seemed to have an intense facial pain. It wore away after I ceased to pay any attention to it.

There is a state of mind and body, not rare in well-developed hysteria, in which there exists a so monstrous development of this strange power to create disorder by thinking of it, that even a slight hint, as it were, will suffice to evoke a novel symptom. In this disease, indeed, we find women, and men too, passing into a mental state in which they are really much like people in dreams. Their power to reason on the phenomena of the senses leaves them, and what they conceive to be the case takes the place of that which is. These are they who are hurt by light, or believe they are; who cannot bear noise, or think they cannot; who feel vibrations as pain; who live muffled lives in dark rooms, and believe they cannot walk, or even lift a hand, or move the head. Such cases are looked upon as simulations of disease by some writers, and are, I am sure, prone to pass into that evil stage of hysteria; but there are others I also know who live lives of odd inhibition—slaves to the tyrant ideas which they themselves create.

This, of course, is to be met with, to some extent, in all grave hysteric cases; but it is also, as I have said, the ruling feature of a few. If you cause such hysteric women as these to believe that you can cure them, you enlist on your side their own troops, for as you can create symptoms, so can you also create absence of symptoms. There is in all this something like the so-called magnetizing of which we used to hear and see so much. Under a fixed belief people were made unable to move, or could not close the eyes, or could not open them, or were made to seem to have a pain by touching a point on the body. The patients I speak of are all very subject to like delusions. You put a finger firmly on the spine, and ask if the patient have now a pain in the left breast? She says no. You persist. At last she says, "Yes— Oh, it hurts me!" Now, is this pure sham, or is it not? Does the presence of the set belief create pain? Is it like the pain of dreams, which seems real enough while we are in the state of dreaming? I have thought over all this a great deal. When we put a finger on the eye unopened for days, and say "Now you can open it," and this is done; or when we arrest motion by an order, we see a plain physical result which must have behind it a ganglionic change out of which it grows; and so it seems to me that, looking at the pain evoked by ideas or beliefs in the light we get from the motor phenomena, so evolved, we are hardly wise to stamp these pains as non-existent.

At the same time that I put forward this doubt as to the justice of the common view, I am far from thinking that the hysteric girl of the class I am now discussing suffers as sharply as she seems to do; the emotions are no more under control than in a dream, and no pains are little, no burdens light.

I have now in my care Miss C. from Milwaukee. When I first saw her she was in bed, which she quit but rarely and with difficulty. The room was kept dark, and she wore blue glasses over the closed eyes, and outside of all a bandage. She used cotton in her ears, and her nurse and parents crept about in list slippers. She had in all ten pillows, large and small,

6

as supports around her, and was, as a young hysterical girl once told me, " crowded with symptoms."

The character of this girl had always been that of a
person thoughtful of and for herself, and not free from
esteem for her own mental powers, so that she had
been able and also very willing by degrees to rule
a meek household with that reckless despotism the
throne of which is very often the couch of an invalid.

This case seemed to me one in which set beliefs,
easily gotten and well nursed, had attained a power
which gave rise to pain and over-sensitiveness and
more or less inhibited movement. I began to deal
with it by learning all I could from the girl herself
to add to what I already knew of her mind, her morals,
her habits, tastes, friends, education, and home life.
Then the talk was left to settle on her eyes, and at
last on the uses of light, and the fact that its excess
hurts even the healthy, but does not injure them.
When at last she grew interested, and with herself
for a text that was easy, I said, that perhaps a woman
of strong character might learn to bear the light after
long disuse of her eyes; that such a one could not get
well readily in the dark, and that although the light
would pain her, it most surely could not cause disease. I then left her, with the idea that she could in
a few days conquer her rebel eyes, and that it was
absurd for a woman of intellect to let one organ disorder the whole body. The next day I found her
with open eyes and sunlight in the room. One by one
the ideas on which the case was built were thus art-
fully removed, and she is now after but a few days of
treatment far on the road to health.

These victories are less easy with older women; but even then the mode of dealing with them is as much a question of the basis of character as of anything else. Sometimes we only need to dispel one symptom to overcome all; sometimes the return to health and healthy ideas exacts a long and tiresome struggle. Sometimes it is safe to assure the patient at the outset that she has but to believe and exert herself in order to walk.

In this infirmary, I saw a few years ago, an abrupt success obtained in this latter way in a woman, fifteen years in bed, who was made able to walk well in three weeks, and I could easily add, were it needed, the details of many other and less striking cases.

I had meant to say something here of that form of hysteria in which the patient deliberately acts a part and with more or less cunning deceives those about her. I have seen a goodly number of these cases, but among them I have found quite rare the attempt to simulate palsy. It is easy enough to learn when a woman is pretending to pass calculi or vomit snake-bones, but to know if her loss of power be real, or if she be suffering from an inhibitory idea or belief is more difficult. I may say, however, that purely simulated palsies in hysterical girls, lack the qualities of hystero-palsies, are too complete, and show no loss of feeling. The best cases I can recall were in very young girls, and were present with much mental disturbance, and after a long role of hysteric symptoms had been played with success.

One of the cases I lately showed you was a curious and most instructive illustration of imitation where distress and terror at witnessing disease in a sister were the efficient factors.

Mary C., aged nine, had frequent, sudden, and severe attacks of epilepsy. After they had lasted two years, the mother brought her to my clinic, and with her a lad aged eleven. He was a puny, feeble, pallid boy, easily alarmed, and so nervous that he could hardly answer my questions. It seemed that nearly six months before I saw him, he ran a nail into his foot, and, about the time the wound healed, had something like an hysterical attack, which seems to have impressed him with the idea that he was afflicted in the same manner as his sister. Soon after this he had what the mother called a spasm, whenever the girl was attacked, and still later when he heard she had a convulsion, or at times without this suggestive cause. His attacks began with tremor. He was said then to become insensible and to shake all over violently. There was no tongue biting, and no coma following the attack, and no facial spasm. After becoming satisfied of the psychical origin of his disorder, I ordered him a cold douche whenever attacked, and directed that he should have the hot iron applied to his neck if the attacks did not cease in a month. At the same time the sister's fits were controlled by bromides, so that he ceased to have before him the constant incitement to attacks. Without further treatment, the boy's fits, if I may so call them, promptly disappeared, not all at once, but by degrees, and he is now well. That in this case the fits of the boy were imitative is clear enough—that without the model before him they would not have arisen is plain.

We need not ask a cause for simpler forms of imitation, as seen in normal functional acts, as when the
micturition of one in a herd of cattle awakens the
idea among the rest and leads all of them to follow
the example. The imitative tendency is a useful part
of our developing powers, but here in cases like that
of this boy, where there are other children, he alone
imitates. Does the terror he only as a timid nervous
lad feels, intensify his imitative faculty, and what
motive is there for yielding to such a tendency? It
may be that there is a certain pleasure in giving way
to instinctive imitative propensities, and moreover we
must all have observed how some sick children enjoy
the important role of being ill, of being coddled and
attended to, and this is especially noticeable in large
families, or in asylums, where usually no one child
receives in health undue attention. Such aids as
these there are, no doubt, to cases of mimicry, while
sometimes the patient's surroundings are to be blamed,
as fastening the disorder or even as giving such information about symptoms as is consciously or not applied to the perfecting of them, the actor receiving as
it were, from a too sympathetic audience, hints which
enable him the better to sustain his part.

Some of you saw but lately the case which sug-
gests these remarks. Here, again, the actor was a lad.
The following details of his case I owe to his physician,
Dr. Benjamin Smith, of Falsington, in this State:—

O. F., æt. 9, had at school a slight chill, and in the
evening thereafter headache and fever; he was well
next day, but was said to have had headache the day

following. At this date the doctor found him suffering from great tenderness at several points of the spinal column. He could not recall having hurt his back, but a few days later declared that he then remembered having fallen so as to strike the back, and that the pain was severe; also, that, on the same day, he had fallen so as to hurt his head. Both falls were said to have taken place on December 25th.

As soon as the tender spine and headache were known to exist, the lad was kept at home and anxiously cared for, while the pain in the head increased and extended at last to the spine. At this date a remarkable dilatation of the pupils was observed, and, the pains increasing, he would lie in bed and rub his head for relief, or have it rubbed. Meanwhile his pulse was not above 80, and did not rise with the presumed increase of pain; nor did he lose appetite.

About the fourteenth day the headache was said to be at its worst, pains arose all over the body, and the muscles of the neck began to be complained of as sore and stiff, while nausea and pretty violent vomiting added to the alarm which his case excited, being set down, despite Dr. Smith's opinion, as an attack of cerebro-spinal meningitis. At this time, after the vomiting ceased. there was a sudden cessation of all the symptoms; but in a few days more his troubles returned, and with dreadful complaint of head- and back-aches, with universal soreness and utter inability to walk, he was at last brought to me for an opinion and for treatment. His case had then lasted five weeks, and was supposed by some physicians and by his relatives to be of a dangerous gravity.

When I saw this lad he was lying in bed, somewhat flushed, but not in a bad condition; his pulse was 85; his breathing 20; his temperature normal. His eyes were bright, and I was struck, as Dr. Smith had been, by the widely dilated pupil. He was constantly declaring that his head hurt him, and it was, as I observed, very notably retracted, the muscles of the neck being stiff and tender. Any effort to flex the head gave rise to tears, remonstrances, and urgent cries of pain. The scalp was everywhere tender and the whole of the erector spinæ masses were also sore, so that the least tap or touch upon them caused him to cry. His legs were gathered up close to his body, and, besides some loudly expressed annoyance when exposed to a bright light, he complained bitterly of the vibrations caused by carriages passing or of the steps of his nurses when they moved across the room.

If, however, he were interested in anything, I found that I could flex the head or touch the spine without causing pain until his attention was recalled to the act. This—with the absence of fever, the calm pulse, the fair appetite, and a certain watchful and furtive expression—led me to believe that he was more or less consciously mimicking disease. As soon as I felt secure in my opinion, I lifted the lad out of bed, and, with severity, ordered him to stand up; he hesitated a moment, and then dropped the flexed limbs under him, lifted his head at a second order, and, as I released him, walked to his bed—a feat which he had been supposed to be utterly unable

to do.   After this there was no trouble; he was kept
out of bed, and, with a rough rubbing daily and a
little urging, was able to play in the garden in three
days and to go home in a week.   His pains, stiff
neck, and tender spine were never heard of after the
first day in the hospital.   I was careful to have him
kept on a farm away from his home for some months.
There has been no relapse.

This case excited great attention, and was the centre
of the too affectionate regards of many relatives.   The
lad became early aware that he was believed to be in
grave danger.   His head and spinal pains were attributed to meningitis and the symptoms discussed in
his hearing.   Only thus can we account for his curious
condition, when, in the face of opposition founded on
his presumably serious state, Dr. Smith brought him
to me.

I saw some years ago a like case in the person of a
young woman who had nursed two cases of cerebro-
spinal meningitis.   Her imitation was admirable and
for some days took in both her own physician and
myself.

Careful use of the thermometer and a rigorous
study of symptoms can alone enable us to avoid such
traps as these.   They illustrate what may occur in
nervous people, under the influence of depressing
agencies and when surrounded by too great sympathy
and by all the information needed to enable them to
act a part.

The lessons which such cases teach us are obvious
enough.   The need for care in discussing symptoms
before nervous women or children, the necessity of

early apprehension of the true state of things in simulated disease, and the wisdom of acting decisively when once we are sure of our ground, are all of them points on which it is hardly needful that I should dwell.

On my return from Europe in October, 1880, I was asked by Dr. Stryker to see in consultation a number of cases at the Church Home for Children, and, as these present the most amazing illustration of mimicked disease I have ever seen, I shall describe them as being the best possible illustration of nearly every point on which I have dwelt. The home is a handsome, wholesome asylum for children, and is situated a few miles from Philadelphia. It contained about 95 girls and but 6 boys. Both the sick and well when I saw them were amply-nourished, and healthy-looking; nor was it possible to find in their home or in their habits any influences which could be credited with giving birth to neurotic tendencies. The diet was good, the hours regular, the play and out-door life sufficient; neither was there in the education given, nor in the religious training, anything with which it was possible to find fault from a medical point of view.

Dr. Stryker gives me in substance the following account: Margaret Trimble, æt. 12, a rosy and sturdy brunette, in admirable health, is one of a neurotic breed, there being in the immediate family two cases of infantile palsy. On September 4th, in the dormitory, when in bed at night, she began to have without known cause, unless it might have been a trifling indigestion, slight convulsive twitches of the arms and legs, with a little numbness of the extremities. This was a matter of a half hour, and she got up well next day. There were no further attacks until the 11th, and thenceforwards they returned daily. At first she was well in the intervals, and slept and went about like the other girls. Her respiration during the attacks was harsh and noisy, and she made at each inspiration a loud crowing noise, much like the breathing in croup. The attacks, rare at first, soon became frequent, and lasted from fifteen minutes to three hours; attention from others inevitably brought them on, even when she was seated and laughing or chatting with her companions. She would then slip down to the floor, and hands, feet, and body would be seized with uncontrollable convulsive motions, so that it was impossible to keep upon her person clothes or bed covering. During an attack she lay on her back, or rolled from side to side, while both arms and legs thrashed the floor with quick and hard blows. The body was lifted from moment to moment, and thrown down again with violence, in a fashion strange to see. Meanwhile, her face was contorted with swiftly changing grimaces, and the tongue thrust out and drawn in, while her head was thumping hard on the floor. Sleep was apt to follow a fit, and there was at times and later in the case, a good deal of choreoid difficulty in moving, or in handling objects; at times the crowing existed alone, and at times the legs became feeble, and she stumbled and fell about.

This child was sent to the Hospital of the University of Pennsylvania, where she remained two months, under the care of my friend, Professor Horatio Wood.

Dr. Musser, the Registrar, sends me his notes, from which I add the following particulars:—

The muscles of the face, neck, eye, and tongue were at this time unaffected by the spasms. While seated she swayed backwards and forwards in clonic spasms. When lying down, her spasms were much as I have described them. There was lack of coördination in all arm and hand movements, but no anæsthesia anywhere. There was tonic spasm of the adductors of the thighs, and in a slight degree of the flexors of the forearms. All movement ceased in sleep. There was no lesion of the eye ground. The urine was normal. There was a slight systolic roughening at the apex of the heart. The usual remedies for chorea having failed, the actual cautery was twice used on the spine, but with no better fortune. Etherization on a full stomach caused vomiting for twenty-four hours, and a permanent relief of all the symptoms. Under careful and systematic training of the muscles, with much urging, and a good deal of scolding, she made finally a complete recovery.

This girl's case was seen by many of her comrades, and not only excited their amusement and curiosity, but led some of them to imitate her "bark," so that they were reproved by the matron for their tricks.

On September 8th, Dr. Stryker being in the home, Kate Nichols, a wholesome looking girl of 10, was brought to him in the nursery, in what seemed at first to be a sharp attack of false croup. She was breathing hard, gasping, crowing, speechless, and wildly clutching at her throat. Her possible relation to the first case was not then understood, and she was treated as if for croup. The trouble persisted all day, and was noted as made worse by noise, or any excitement, and to be by and by associated with slight convulsive jerkings of the limbs. Meanwhile, the pulse was rapid, but there was no fever. The following night all of these troubles passed away in a sound sleep, from which she awakened crowing and barking· and after a day of increasing nervous agitation, exploded in a convulsion, identical in character with that of case No. 1. The attacks thereafter increased in violence, but all of her functions were well performed. She ate, drank, and passed urine and feces as usual, and when free from convulsions was merry and pleasant, until the approach of a nurse with medicine, or the visit of a manager to the Infirmary, started her off anew. From the outset she began to lose power in the limbs. When held up she would start fairly, but instantly the legs became convulsed, the feet tripped one over the other, and she fell in a fit on the floor.

The girl was also treated at the University much as the last case; the cautery was of little use, but the effect produced by ether on her comrade had a decidedly good moral influence, and seemed to have a good deal to do with her recovery

Case 3.—On September 9th, Sallie Speer was seized with the same form of respiratory spasm, but with the crowing noise there was a continuous chattering of the teeth, like that of a bad ague chill. On the 10th the usual convulsions came on, she having ample preparation from seeing those of the other children. In a few days all of her symptoms passed away, and she returned to the school-room, for a week, when the same disorders reappeared, and she was once more placed in the nursery.

Case 4.—Florence Pierce, æt. 12, had about the 11th like attacks, but, besides the usual convulsions, she had remarkable mydriasis in the intervals. While yet able to walk she had singular attacks of festination, and if going towards her bed would run furiously and be thrown headlong across it, and on to the floor beyond. Generally she crawled about on her hands and knees, with her head swaying about as if it was held up with difficulty.

Case 5.—Miriam Drinkhouse, æt. 11, was depressed on account of having been placed in a lower class than her comrades, owing to her inability to keep up with them in their studies. Next day she was unable to stand, and her first fit followed on October 13th.

Case 6.—Fannie Clark, æt. 12, was taken ill with respiratory spasms, and the same convulsions about October 13th. She had also remarkable coldness of feet and hands, which was not observed in the others.

Florence Mack, æt. 8, Sarah Nolen, æt. 12, Florence Mulligan, æt. 10, Bella Burk, æt. 11, Mary Mitchell, æt. 12, were all taken about the 12th to the 15th of October. Their symptoms were much the same as those above described. There were also a number of other cases, some slight and some severe. Owing to want of space all the first cases were placed in the two adjoining rooms of the infirmary. Here they were seen by one another, and also more or less by such girls as were engaged in the housework. Other cases were soon added, and at last there were at least ten cases in the apartments mentioned. The results of this companionship may be easily imagined; at first the convulsions were irregular as to time, but after awhile they took place only in the evening, and later still in the morning and the evening; although at any time a visit such as mine, or that of Dr. Stryker, or of a lady manager was sufficient to start the attacks. Then one girl would begin to bark or twitch, then a second and a third, until on bed or floor, or seated, ten or twelve children were wheezing, barking, grunting, crowing, or in violent convulsions; while the bewildered nurses ran from one to another, presenting a scene quite astonishing to witness.

During a few days there were many interesting variations in this singular malady. On one occasion, all of the children in the sick ward got out of bed at night, and took to walking about on their hands and knees; at other times some of them described in soliloquy dreams, one saw black men, another, whose mother had been recently pregnant, described herself as having had a child, and mentioned the luxuries she considered desirable for a person so situated. More commonly the girls were scared, or said they were, by wild beasts, and one child would adopt the vision which another related within her hearing. After consultation all of the cases were scattered about among different hospitals,[1] where, as a rule, they made prompt recoveries, under somewhat various treatments. The cases lasted from one month to three.

---

[1] The Jefferson College, the Presbyterian, and the Episcopal Hospitals. I am indebted to Dr. Starr for full notes of several of the cases.

LECTURE IV.

MIMICRY OF DISEASE.

THE cases with which I have illustrated this sub-jcet of mimicry of disease have been, so far, some-what simple and uncomplicated; nor could they have readily or long deceived any watchful physician who had had any experience of neurotic maladies. There are, however, more complicated cases to be met with, and some of these are remote from those so far de-scribed, in that the symptoms were not imitated from models ready at hand, or wholly learned from gabbling nurses or relatives.

They exhibit also the curious progress from simu-lation, not consciously imitative to conscious unre-sisted simulation, and at last dissimulation. I shall relate here two admirable instances of these inter-esting combinations of mimicry passing into well-sustained fraud.

A good many years ago I saw, one evening, a girl, aged 13 years, who had never had any of the maladies of childhood excepting measles. When her new trou-bles began she was not as yet menstruating, nor did she show any notable signs of womanly development.

In January, 1866, when skating, her right instep became chafed severely, and for this she was kept at rest for two or three weeks, but received very little

care from her mother, and, in fact, needed but little.
One day an attack of indigestion ended in vomiting,
which was very violent, and which brought about her
all the sympathy her elder relatives could give. From
this time her appetite failed, and the vomiting recurred at intervals. Long after, she told me that she
could have vomited less, but that everybody was kind
when she was so sick. Here, at least, was a distinct
failure to resist, and probably a desire to aid, in producing sickness of stomach. The vomiting grew more
frequent in the spring, and after a fortnight of fever,
which she is said to have had in June, 1866, all food
was thrown up, and the bowels were opened only
once in ten days, or even less often. These conditions
persisted through 1866, with little change, the child
rejecting everything, and growing at last sallow, and
desperately wasted. The skin became sensitive to
touch, so that no water could be used for fear of causing convulsions, and most of the time she was shaken
by violent hiccough.

The vomiting, at first accidental, was thus at last
aided and cherished for a purpose, until, as often happens, the morbid act became habitual and despotic.
But in a nervous system such as this child's no such
habit could persist without giving rise to other symptoms as grave, while these in turn would be nursed
and developed to win and keep up the sympathy,
attention, and importance, which are among the unnatural moral appetites, of a nature once started upon
this disastrous road so strewn with multiple disorders. When such persons get well, their lips are
so surely sealed by shame and self-disgust, as to make

it difficult to verify by frank confession the suspicions which arose in the minds of bystanders, or to trace the fatal steps by which the victim descends, from the state in which she welcomes a symptom, to the degradation of creating symptoms. My patient, when first seen by me, had been abandoned, as in a dying state, by two homœopathic physicians, who had left for her use a prescription of rather ample doses of morphia.

The picture which this child presented when first I saw her was not readily to be forgotten. She was lying on her back, staring upwards, with glassy eyes set deep in dark rings, which faded into a sallow leathery skin, drawn tense over projecting bones. Her mouth was wide open, the jaw dropped, and the whole cavity literally lined with thrush (muguet).[1] The skin of the body was dry, and splotched with islets of dusky red, and the bedclothes were kept off of the sensitive surface by a shelter of half-hoops. As I stood and looked at this singular spectacle, apparently that of a dying child, she groaned at brief intervals, and also coughed a good deal, at such times expressing pain in her face, but usually lying quite still, with a look of merely the most profound melancholy. A careful study enabled me to find no organic disease. Her urine was so scanty that she often passed but two ounces a day; but this was not albuminous; the belly was very tender to touch, although, if I distracted her attention, neither touch nor pressure caused any sign of pain; attention was needful to enable her to feel these pains, but as it may be said that attention is for

---

[1] The coating of *oidium albicans* was the most remarkable I have ever seen.

all pain a reinforcing element, too much stress must not be laid on this point. I noticed, however, that this wretched, wilted, starved creature followed my motions with attentive eyes, although she never turned her head.

I asked for milk, and put within her lips a table-spoonful, for which she closed her mouth; a moment passed, and with a gulp she threw it up. I repeated the dose, keeping a finger on the larynx. Again she threw up, or seemed to; for, as the larynx did not make the usual upward movement which accompanies the act of deglutition, it was clear that she had not swallowed at all. I watched this neat little fraud several times. Usually she swallowed a part of each mouthful, and, holding the rest in her mouth, suddenly cast it out with a very fair imitation of the convulsive act of emesis. When quite sure of having correctly observed her, I abruptly charged her with the deceit. At first she denied in a faint voice, and saying she couldn't help it, began to cry. A little sternness enabled me to get down her a full glass of milk. I then cleared the room of all her friends, threw away the hoops, and sat down by her side. She was evidently conquered and alarmed, which I did not wish her to be. I therefore took her hand quietly, and told her that she could get well; that milk was needful; that, if thrown up, it would be given again, and that I meant to feed her whether she liked it or not.

The after-care, which owed its success largely to the care of Dr. Wm. W. Keen, was arduous enough. The belly—and, indeed, the whole skin—was rubbed twice a day with sweet oil; milk was given freely and often, and the bowels rid of their packed contents by the use of frequent enemata. I found the spine exquisitely tender, but, as is often the case, this was much helped by ice-bags (dry cold). Meanwhile the thrush faded under the use of washes of sulphite of soda. The patient's head was elevated a little day by day, and the diet was increased and varied. The bowels proved so obstinate that nothing but croton oil moved them, and the trouble of swallowing persisted for some time, although lessened whenever her attention could be called away from the act of deglutition. Incessant attention to the muscular apparatus of the throat had made the use of these parts difficult, and swallowing having ceased to be automatic, was re-embarrassed by every new concentration upon it of an act of will. When she received milk in her mouth it always rested there for some time; if, however, the head was thrown back, and at the same time the larynx pushed up by a hand, this sort of hint usually proved successful, and the movement of deglutition was completed. By degrees this trouble passed away, and she gained in strength so as to sit up, and after awhile to stand.

The use of induction currents to the disused muscles was a further help, and, with the gain in power, came back easier movements of bowels and bladder, and a more wholesome moral tone. Within six weeks the girl was able to call at my house, and she is now I believe, the healthy mother of a family.

I could never extract from this child, when well, anything beyond the statement that she "just could not help it;" and if I pressed her further, she said she was sorry, and took refuge in tears.

About two years ago I saw, with Dr. Finn, a case quite as remarkable. The girl, aged thirteen years, living in Ohio, after an attack of ague, began to limp a little one day, and said she had a pain in the right knee. A physician examined it, and told her parents quite truly that there was no cause for alarm, advising at the same time exercise, and a let-alone treatment. This would have answered well, and have saved much trouble, had not some one persuaded her mother to ask advice of the travelling agent of a surgical institute, who diagnosed hip-joint disease, put on a temporary splint, and arranged to cure the child at the institute. From this time, when the little public opinion about the girl pronounced for a grave malady, she grew speedily worse, and under the influence of the discussions as to the hip-joint disease and its symptoms, she began to act out as fully as possible the pathological drama so foolishly taught her. The pain increased, and the leg contracted at the knee and hip. At the institute things grew worse, and very soon there was double hip disease, and local applications, and splints, many and wonderful. But when one of these curious cases is well engaged in this career of simulation, there comes a time when, either because the first trouble no longer excites sympathy, or for more complex reasons, these forms of disease become progressive and invasive. In our little patient, the contractions of the thigh remaining, the arms, especially the left, became flexed, the feet being in full extension. At this time hysterical spasms came on; the eyelids closed, and remained shut; and, most strange of all, she was unable to eat before 9 o'clock P. M. In this state the child was first seen by Dr. Finn, who removed her to quiet lodgings, where soon afterwards I saw her, and heard this exasperating history of folly and quackery. As I first saw her, she lay on the bed, her back to the light—a queer little shrivelled creature, tawny of tint, and the skin covered with bran-like scales, washing being a rare ceremony. Legs and arms were drawn up so as almost to hide the thin, ancient-looking and cunning little visage, which seemed so blind with its closed but quivering lids, and yet so unnaturally astute in its intentness of attention when her own case was mentioned or discussed.

Her right hip was red and swollen, and the thumbs of both hands had been so long and tightly contracted as to have caused the palms to ulcerate, while the whole skin was sensitive to such a degree that the bedclothes were not allowed to touch her, and she uttered a muffled cry of dismay and seeming terror at every approach; her voice was reduced to a faint whisper, and she was said to be totally blind.

The treatment in this case was of easy enough application in a child. A single nurse was left in charge. The legs were violently straightened and their owner invited to set them in order, so as to avoid in future this abrupt and painful treatment. We were told as usual that she never could eat until nine P. M., and wonder was expressed that, having her eyes shut, she was able to know what o'clock it was. The clock on the mantel was an obvious aid, and at all events, when set forward two hours, the nine o'clock meal was asked for at seven. The gain in this case was steady and easy enough. I lost sight of the child after she left us to return home, but at the time of her departure she was nearly well, and, I learn, has entirely recovered.

I have often thought that, if I could induce older patients who had been affected more or less like these children to relate to me their histories with sufficient frankness, I should obtain a larger insight into the motives which prompt them to cultivate or to create symptoms. As interesting additions to this rare branch of medical autobiography the three letters which I subjoin must suffice :—

"The period of my life about which you ask me, I can only look back upon with a sort of disgust which makes it unpleasant for me to speak about ; it is only the hope that some one else may be helped by it which makes me willing to speak of it at all. I was brought up by an invalid aunt, and I often think of what you once said to me, that the women who indulge their own nervous systems are those who most indulge children. My aunt taught me very early to notice and dwell upon any little symptom I happened to have, and, when I was fourteen, I un-luckily hurt my knee. For this I was kept in bed two weeks, and, when I wanted to get up, I was told to keep quiet. Under this enforced rest my appetite failed, and I began to have nausea. My first vomit-ing created a sensation in the household, which I think, as I recall it, I enjoyed as making me impor-tant. Very soon I got to vomiting every day ; there was none of the nausea which I had at first, and which I have since been familiar with as a part of sea-sickness. It gave me no annoyance to cast up my food, and was indeed rather a relief. From this time I was surrounded with sympathy and doctors. A few months later my aunt died and I was left in charge of an uncle and aunt, and became one of a large circle of children, among whom I got very little of the care which had before this encompassed me. I remember well that I resented the change, and, finding that if I took little food I excited alarm, I began to yield to the tendency to excite distress and anxiety by taking little or no food at times. I suppose this abstinence gave rise to the nervousness, and finally to the spasms which came on at this time, at least I can give no further explanation; I only know that every new symptom caused new anxiety, and that I somehow liked it all. After a while a new doctor was called in, and under his rule, which was very stern, I got better, and was able to leave home and go to the seashore, where, under new influences and interests, I lost all of my symptoms except the vomiting, which seemed to me uncontrollable. I lost this only by resolute efforts; in fact, by efforts so desperate that often, when food rose in my mouth, I swallowed it again. I do not think I should ever have so tried if I had not overheard a person in whom I had a great interest express himself as having heard with disgust of my habit. Then, as you know, I learned from you that the habit could be broken; I succeeded, as you know, and am married and have a little girl, and I can promise you that she at least will never be allowed to go through what I have done."

I presume that this partial self-analysis is as near to a full and truthful statement of the motives which urge to mimetic fraud as we are likely to get. I have been told by one woman that she was as irresponsible as one in a dream; while more usually you are told simply "I do not know why I did it; I could not have meant to deceive any one." My next extract from these confessions is in some sense honest enough, and, as I said before, is curious, both as to what it reveals and what it hides. The writer is long since dead, and I am therefore at liberty to use her letter with such precautions as make identification impossible.

I had seen my patient in the morning and received this letter in the evening. For several weeks she had been under my care with these conditions, a good rosy color, fair weight, and regular functions; but at times enormous losses of urine and intense spinal irritability, which forbade her to stand or to walk a step. For her food she ate a chop at breakfast, and no other food the rest of the day. You must not understand me to say that I accepted all these statements, but merely as briefly sketching what seemed to be her state. This very pretty invalid was a charming and witty, and most accomplished person. After her husband's death, she had taken to her couch, and, despite aches and ailments, was in her becoming sick outfit the centre of an attractive circle, which gladly gathered about the couch, on which she was carried from room to room. I hardly know under what circumstances she developed the full range of her powers. The irritable spine came first, and as one doctor after another was consulted other symptoms were added to her repertory.

She had been some little while under my care when I saw two things which confirmed my well-grounded suspicions as to the nature of her case; she slept alone, disliking the constant presence of a nurse · but she rarely failed to ring for her attendant twice every night.

The last morning I saw her I had occasion to look at her feet, and noticed that her soles were dotted with black marks; coupling this with the fact that she had complained of her wood fire as having smoked, I concluded that she had been afoot in the night, and that the dark marks came from "blacks" on the floor, the result of a defective fire draught. A moment later, observing some crumbs on her bolster, I asked her to sit up that I might examine her spine. As she rose, I threw aside her pillow, and saw under it two oranges, several slices of bread, and a banana. To my amazement she said coolly, "Well, now I am caught; I thought you would do it soon or late." My rather sharp remonstrances seemed only to amuse her, and that evening I received the letter, a part of which I print.

"Before this reaches you I shall have made arrangements to leave. The game I have played on you I have played on others, and in my restricted life I have found it very amusing. You must not blame my maid, as I paid the woman who cleaned the room to bring me food. I found that doctors got tired of my sore back, and that they ceased to feel interest in me, a thing I never did like, so I began to complain of queer symptoms, and as this often aroused new interest, I went on experimenting until I hit on the starvation idea, which has done very well; of course I got up at nights and walked a good deal too, but how you knew it I would like to know. As to the urine, I used to fill up the vessel with water. I hope you will not tell my doctor at home, you would take away a good deal that is pleasant, and spoil an interesting case too."

These are the only cases of this form of moral obliquity, in which I have ever been able to get a free confession. They expose, I fancy, to some extent, the motives which underlie the duplicity of such women.

The last of these statements is more recent, and I have permission to print it. It is in some ways more valuable than the others; the belief this woman at last reached as to the want of foundation for her presumed physical disabilities, and her continued conviction that the pains were as distinct as any pain, must, I think, be received with respect. I am sure that she has done her best to analyze her symptoms truthfully.

She came to me on a couch, or litter, from a Western State, a girl of 19, not wasted, and of good tints. She was said to be unable to walk, motion hurt her; and her eyes were carefully guarded from light by a double bandage. She was kindly but firmly treated, and was able in a few days to bear sunlight, and to go downstairs. When once she had been made sure that all this could be done without death, I allowed her to go forward more slowly, with such help from tonics, good diet, etc., as I could give. She very often talked to me about the cause for her disorder, and out of my inquiries and interest in her case came the self-analysis I append. It needs no commentary.

"I suppose, in all cases of nervous affections, one's natural temperament and constitution play an important part, and, doubtless, with me, a temperament rather emotional, sensitive, and occasionally morbid, had something to do with making possible the state I was in when I went to see Dr. Mitchell, in December, 1879.

"The immediate cause for the headaches, which began a year before that time and never left me after it, seemed to be a few weeks of mental and social strain. I had for two years before that time suffered from a weak back, had felt constantly tired, spent much of my time on the bed, and taken but little exercise. But in the fall of 1878 I felt much better and undertook study and class recitation, and became much interested in some evening literary and social clubs. For a few weeks I went every day to the utmost limit of my strength, and was then suddenly prostrated with severe headache and excessive weariness.

"I, of course, tried quiet and rest immediately, and after a while grew better, but had a return of headache and weariness whenever I tried exerting myself much again. There is no question that what I lacked then was courage. If some one could have told me that there was nothing of consequence the matter, I am sure I should have overcome the difficulty and very soon have gained endurance by exertion; but, instead, I became afraid to do things for fear of bringing suffering, and, as month after month passed, I could do less and less. I cannot now understand why I could not have seen, why I could not realize that the less I did the less I could do; but I was blind, and so was every one else. I thought it was some strange, mysterious disease that was taking away my strength. By summer, a few minutes' conversation or the walk of a block would make the pain in my head agonizing, and every sound became unendurable. My eyes, too, shared in my good-for-nothing state.

"In the fall, the pain went into my back and limbs and sent me to bed with the strange infatuation that I could not move without injury, as I certainly could not without pain. I had lain in one position with closed eyes for eight weeks, before going to Dr. Mitchell, in a state of supposed helplessness. One thing I want to say in extenuation of myself, and that is that the pain was real, not fancied. Whatever its cause or however easily it might have been averted, it was genuine suffering at the time. I was scarcely ever hysterical either in the usual sense of the term, for, at least, I realized the necessity of self-control.

"In looking back over that year with the light of the present, I can only say that I believe there was nothing really the matter with me, only it seemed as if there was, and, because of those sensations, I carried on a sort of starvation process, physical and mental. Why that process should have brought me into such a condition, I must leave with some one wiser than I

LECTURE V.

UNUSUAL FORMS OF SPASMODIC AFFECTIONS IN WOMEN.

You will find, if you come to have much experience in the cases of hysterical women, that in some instances the disorder arises in general convulsions following upon a state of acquired nervous instability, and then runs on into a great variety of symptoms—palsies, hyperæsthesias, and anæsthesias, and contractions—to end, at last, in years of bed-ridden invalidism, or, much more rarely, in spinal sclerosis. A single case will thus give you, in disorderly and unexpected succession, every scene of what I have ventured elsewhere to call the drama of hysteria.

At the risk of repeating an old story, I have sought, in one of these lessons, to relate some of these histories, chiefly that I might illustrate afresh the termination in sclerosis, and partly to show what might be done to rescue certain of what seem to be the most hopeless of these exasperating cases.

Apart from these, however, we see two forms of hysterical disorder, in which the primary signs are either slight and aborted, or remain so inconspicuous as to give but little aid in the early diagnosis. One of these is marked by mental derangements, and is usually treated as simply a causeless insanity until

8*

some outbreak of the commoner forms of hysteric signs reveals the true condition. I mention it here only to complete my rather rude and partial classification. The other is characterized by the extraordinary variety and strangeness of the convulsive disorders, which, for years, and from time to time, afflict the patient; all other symptoms being present rarely, or in feebly-represented forms. I propose to relate and discuss for you some of the most unusual of these cases.

In 1871 I was consulted by an intelligent unmarried lady, Miss L. P., æt. 26, from Mississippi, for a condition of system which was probably due to certain emotional disturbances following a violent onset of cholera morbus. The attack was repeated a few days later. The day after, she had intense burning pain between the shoulders and down the whole length of the spine. This symptom lasted long, and with it, for a month, during which she kept her bed, there were brief periods of febrile activity. She is said to have had no severe headache, and no uterine or urinary symptoms. On first rising she found that her legs were feeble, and this paresis was best marked on the left side.

When first seen by me these symptoms remained unchanged. The weakness of the left side was complained of both in the arm and leg, and as affecting the eye. She needed a supporting arm when walking, but did as well in the darkness as in the light, and stood fairly well with shut eyes. The left sole was slightly less sensitive than the right. Above this there was no dysæsthesia. There was also no analgesia, and

heat and cold were well distinguished. There was, at
times, a sense of extreme weight on the chest. The
burning pain in the spine was unequally distributed.
It was worse at the 5th and 6th dorsal vertebræ, and
was increased at night and by fatigue. The temporary
application of ice made it worse, and this increased suf-
ering was felt for some time afterwards. Elsewhere she
had no fixed suffering, but complained of darting neuralgic pains almost at any point of the body. There
was no womb trouble of moment. On the left side there
was a large area of variable iliac tenderness, not great,
and sometimes absent. It was less on deep pressure
than on slight touch. The eye-grounds were normal,
but she was said to have at times double vision, if
very tired.

This case, as I recall it, puzzled me greatly, and
was finally treated as of organic cerebro-spinal
origin; and this idea was strengthened by the fact
that at times there was distinct rigidity of the erector spinæ muscles. She came under my care first in
the autumn of 1872, and gradually improved. The
back was several times cauterized early in January,
1873, and great gain followed. Somewhat later a slight
and singular tottering of gait was seen; but, on the
whole, the progress was good and steady; so that, by
the end of January, 1874, she could walk with ease a
quarter of a mile on level ground. In February,
1874, Miss P. made the mistake of leaving home,
and subjecting herself to what was, for her, excessive
fatigue and much social excitement. Then, as always
since, fatigue brought on more or less nervousness,
and the singular forms of spasms which have proved

so enduring an annoyance. At the close of a day of unusual fatigue, on rising from her chair to cross the room, she suddenly staggered back, and then rotated violently several times. These fits returned over and over, and resulted within a week in fresh dorsal pain, extreme lassitude, and a curious inability to keep her balance. Meanwhile, the rotations were usually, but not always, to the left. The loss of equilibrium was great. On rising she would pitch forward, and then sideways, and then turn swiftly. The pitching was really convulsive, and not due to lack of balancing power, and there was no subjective sense of giddiness. She came to see me soon after, and was much worse for the journey. During ten days of quiet here the rotatory spasms gave place to violent and nearly constant spasmodic jerking of the head backwards or forwards, to right or to left. As this also departed she had a new onset of what she called "twists," and thenceforward turned only to the left. These spasms were amazing things to see—suddenly, while crossing the room, she would rotate furiously to the left—about three to six times. The turn was very rapid, and seemed to begin with the spine. Then the head followed, and, as she said, it seemed hard for the legs to keep up with the back.

At other times an irresistible power seemed to drag her up on to her tiptoes, where she would remain a moment, as it were, fixed. At this time she could walk, or even run backwards, but a forward movement was beset with difficulties. She would be, as it were, hurled forward, and then rotate, or the effort to move in a forward direction would end in a rapid retrogressive stagger, followed by rotation to left.

There was no vertigo except as a result of the spin-
ning. In June she went home, and from this period
she had a succession of slow gains with sudden relapses. If leading a very quiet life, she sometimes
passed six months without spasms. Worry, fatigue,
excitement were all sure to bring them on. At times
there was no warning, but usually pain in the feebler
leg, nervousness and irritability were premonitory of
an attack. Then she would of a sudden find one leg
oddly twisted around the other, or would be drawn
up on to her toes, or forced to walk on her heels, or
would pitch hither and thither, not from weakness,
but from alternating unilateral spasms. At these times
her will seemed to be absolutely suspended. "It is,"
she says, "as if some other will power had me in
possession. I struggle against it in vain."[1]

The first point to notice in this case is its generic
relation to the class of functional spasms of Duchenne;
those in which spastic movements are associated with
or follow some form of normal muscular action.
Such spasms do not arise during repose, and in this
sense chorea is at first, and in some cases throughout,
as I have elsewhere observed, a form of functional
spasm.[2] Perhaps I shall, in a measure, clear your
minds as to the nature of what I mean by functional
spasms if I recall to you the influence of strychnia in
large doses—such as you have seen given here many
times. You will remember that in certain spinal

[1] For analogous cases see Russell Reynolds's System of Medicine,
art. Chorea.

[2] Am. Journ. Med. Sci., October, 1876.

maladies, such as those of syphilitic birth, it is my habit first to give iodides in heavy doses, and then to suspend these for a time, and to give strychnia up to the limit of physiological endurance, that is to say, until I cause an approach to spasms. When, for example, you give hypodermically the one-fifth to the one-eighth of a grain daily—the patient will have little or no annoyance if you are careful to insist that he remain at absolute rest in bed for two hours after each injection. If there be any tendency to spastic twitchings of the muscles, the will is competent to control them, unless, and this is the point I would make, the patient attempts to exercise. Should he do this, the effort results at once in irregular movements of an incoördinate character, and in slight or more grave spasms of the muscles employed. While at rest there is no obvious trouble, but voluntary movement occasions spasms, which are the offspring of the poison. They are, in a word, functional spasms, and would not be seen at all, with limited use of strychnia, were it not for the efforts at voluntary action.

The second consideration to which it is worth while to call attention was the great variety of the forms assumed by Miss L. P.'s attacks, and the temporary limitation of the disorder to partial groups of muscles. This alone would, I think, entitle us to suspect hysteria as a cause; and, when we learn that no attacks ever took place in the street, and that pleasant surroundings lessened the likelihood of the occurrence of the spasms, while all depressing and enfeebling agencies were apt to bring them on, no further doubt should exist as to the parentage of the disorder. Muscular action perfect in health loses in force and in sureness, and in steadiness, as any one falls away from the highest standard of physical condition, and when there is in the ganglia some cause tending towards irregularity in any shape, it also is apt to rise into gravity just in proportion to the failure in physical status. Add to this emotional disturbances, which in certain natures are prone to express themselves in some form of irregular muscular acts, and we have all the needed factors for producing such convulsions in persons at all capable of evolving them.

I consider that the treatment, which I need not here consider, utterly failed. I never succeeded in raising my patient's health to such a level as to put her above the possibility of these curious attacks. I, perhaps, ought rather to say that I never could keep her at that level. The least blow to health was with her a knock down, and recovery was slow. Practically speaking, the woman who habitually has hysterical spasms has something wrong with her general health. She is anæmic, or has lost general tone, and cannot get up, so to speak, or there is that remarkable state of easy tire which is called nervous exhaustion, but which were often better called nervous exhaustibility, and which is, perhaps, due to some form of defective nutrition of the nerve centres. Always there is some such cause behind the spasms. If we can relieve it we cure the convulsions, or rather make the soil fatal to their growth. I do not think this is always possible. There are some anæmias which resist all treat-

ment.   There are some mysterious forms of nutritive
failure which are never made well.

I have seen recently a case which somewhat resembles Miss L. P.'s.   Miss C., a native of Maryland,
æt. 21, was sent, when 17 years old, to a school in
which boys and girls were educated together.   Just
before leaving home she had two slight attacks of
"stiffness" when rising from the sitting posture.
While at school she never menstruated, although
previously regular.   Next came a light attack of
diphtheria, and still her general health seems not to
have been obviously damaged ; but the "contractions
grew more frequent until at last one day, in class, she
was unable to speak, owing to trismus which came
on as she rose to recite.   She went home after this
event, and in a few weeks her menstrual flow returned; nevertheless the spasms continued, and this
despite a gradual rise in health, and a nature free
from melancholy, and prone to seek and find healthy
enjoyment in outdoor life.   A further gain followed
a residence of some weeks in the West, but still the
attacks continued ; nor did it seem that almost perfect health secured immunity.

At present, in 1880, this young woman looks in admirable condition ; nor is there, on careful study of her
case, any evidence of organic disease or functional disorder.   While seated she never has any symptom of
spasm ; but many times in each day, when rising from
a seated or recumbent posture, she is seized with attacks which I have now seen her exhibit many times.

On rising she is seized with spasms of the legs,
neck, face, and arms and hands.   These vary end-

lessly, and are not often exactly alike in any two attacks. Usually the phenomena are these, and in this order :—

Just as she begins to move, after rising from a chair, she has—

1. A stiffening of the muscles of the legs and chiefly of those of the thighs. This causes a certain constraint in her first steps, but does not prevent them.

Having moved a few steps she has—

2. A consentaneous spasm of the neck (twist to left and downward pull), of the body, also to left, of the lower part of the face, either to left or right, or stiffness from bilateral spasm of face. The left arm is sometimes in violent flexion from fingers to shoulder, or the arm is extended and the hand flexed. There is the same variety as to the movements of the right arm. When I last saw a fit the right arm and hand were thrown out in rigid extension, the left being as perfectly in flexion.

3. No matter what posture was assumed, she was so to speak, fixed in it for perhaps ten to fifteen seconds. The spasm came on, and rather slowly culminated in some one odd posture, and there and then the woman became, as it were, a statue for the moments that followed.

4. These spasms were painless, and disappeared in an instant.

5. They caused no confusion, or vertigo, or any other ill feeling, nor any sleepiness. She went on at once to do whatever she had meant, such as to walk or to dance.

9

At times the attacks are frequent, at others rare, and absence from home and change of scene and climate seem to lessen the number of fits.

6. These spasms are often but not always preceded by a condition which is sometimes chronic, at others comes only as an immediate warning of attack; at all events its presence is a sure sign that the attacks will come on readily and be more than commonly hard to prevent. This precedent state consists in a slight general tingling which varies in amount, and is apt to be accompanied by a sense of stiffness in the muscles of the legs. These are rather evidences of a chronic and slight condition of spasm than of anything which it is worth while to call an aura.

If, on rising, she stands still a moment and prepares herself to walk by some indescribable mental act, which is not a mere resolve because here the will is quite powerless, she can prevent an attack. To rise quickly and walk at once, or to turn abruptly just after beginning to walk are apt to cause fits.

The relationship of such attacks of functional spasm as these is as near to chorea as to epilepsy, for the state of which she speaks as favoring and preceding a fit cannot for reasons already given be looked upon as an aura, and we know of no epilepsies in which the functional and orderly act of a muscle or muscles gives rise in some way to the irregular and disorderly discharge of nerve force which constitutes a spasm. But in grave chorea, this is precisely what does occur, the forms of spasm having of course in that disorder, as in functional spasms, differentiating peculiarities. I gave this woman bromide of lithium chiefly to see if the bromides would control or lessen the fits. The attacks were not lessened by this agent.

After this failure I was at a loss how to deal with the case. There are spasms which are so nearly a part of the normal muscle acts or so tied up with them as to be as hard to change by medicine as the orderly sequence of any common muscular action, nor is the task of reform more easy when years of repetition have made deep the easy ruts of habit. I could only insist that she must live so careful a life as never to rise without being on guard. Then also, since violent exertion distinctly lessened her tendency to spasms, I advised an abundance of exercise. The results of this advice were good, and the case rapidly prospered when she took to hard housework, which happened to interest her very greatly.

The next case which I desire to add to this group of spasmodic disorders, is, like the last two, remarkable for the great variety of distorting forms assumed in turn. Some of you may recall the patient, a poor unmarried seamstress, aged forty-three, tall, thin, and with a face constantly and deeply flushed; a pulse of 90 to 100, and, so far as I could discover, no organic disease. When nearing the age of forty she began to have retarded menstrual flow, but neither then nor when seen by me a year later, was there any uterine trouble. In June, 1878, after some family annoyances, she had a severe rigor, ending in trismus which came on abruptly, and repeated itself thereafter with like suddenness, and at inconvenient seasons, usually while she was eating. In August it was replaced by dysphagia. She acquired, as a consequence of this condition, a deadly fear of the abortive efforts to swallow, and would chew for many minutes before making an attempt at deglutition. In the autumn this too passed away, and in October she first consulted me at my clinic for a "lump" on the chest. I was about to refer her to one of our surgeons when her remark that it went and came interested me, and I carefully examined it. To my surprise the growth was in or on the left great pectoral above the breast. It was an oval flattened swelling with quite abrupt edges. If I carried the arm out so as to make the muscle tense, in a few minutes the tumor disappeared gradually, and I perceived that it was a phantom tumor with which I had to deal. I was familiar enough with these as seen in or on the belly, but I now saw only my second case of this phenomenon in any other muscular mass. The "tumor" was hard and dense, and the temperature over it was a half degree above that of the neighboring parts. Hard rubbing gradually dispersed it, but it formed again in a few hours, and I may add was always tender.

I next found to my great interest that all of the pectoral on this side was in a state of curious irritability, and this you will recognize as only an increase of a normal quality. When, for example, I strike a healthy muscle with a finger tip, or better, a pointed caoutchouc percussion-hammer, such as that which we use to test tendon reflexes—two facts are observable. First, the whole length of the muscular fibre struck contracts, or a large part of the whole length. Then, as it relaxes, a little hard prominence forms in the muscle at the part struck, and remains for a few seconds until it gradually disappears.[1] In this woman's case, the secondary local contraction was larger than is usual, and lasted for at least a half hour or more. A few weeks later, she came to the hospital to stay, and now the pectoral tumor had gone, and the belly presented the usual appearance of a phantom tumor. All of its muscles were violently contracted, so as to look like a rounded growth. It was painfully tender and the percussion note was dull. It, however, presented one peculiarity I had never seen in any other such case. Several times a day the whole contraction passed away, but the least handling of the belly brought it all back, or this took place without any interference. The woman was during all this time in a state of amazing nervousness, and was seized with universal tremor whenever any one came near to her bed. Her pulse rose at times to 130, and the temperature fluctuated daily and irregularly from 97° F. to 105° F. We got her well enough to walk about and to leave the hospital, but the abdominal contraction still existed or did so after a year had passed away.

I have seen a similar false tumor in the calf of a highly hysterical lady. It was relieved in a week or two by the daily use of massage.

I shall complete this group of cases by a very singular one, which I saw last year. M. B., female, æt. 59, a worn-out school teacher, always feeble and lacking blood, but otherwise well, had a slight sprain of the

---

[1] I described these phenomena many years ago in the Trans. of the Phila. Acad. Nat. Sci., not then being aware that Weber had called attention to them. They are best seen in the pectorals of thin people.

knee, which forced her to remain at rest. Very soon she perceived a rhythmical spasm of the middle of the muscular masses of the calf of the left leg. The muscle gathered into a hard painful swelling about five inches below the popliteal space. The contraction, which was two by three and one-half inches in size, was sudden and horribly painful, and the region attacked was always sore, but was most so during the spasm. This lasted a few seconds, but the space affected was at all times hot and a little hard. The spasms were singularly regular, about twenty-five to thirty a minute, but there were often long periods of one to five hours during which no spasm existed. She had been treated in various ways without relief, but I was finally enabled to help her by rest in bed, the use of a splint, and careful feeding and iron, but the local trouble was not entirely cured until I had used several injections of atropine, which were thrown into the muscle, a plan which was, I think, first employed by Drs. Morehouse, Keen, and myself in the Hospital for Nervous Diseases during our civil war.

To complete the group of unusual forms of spasm in women, I shall only add a case or two of hysterical athetosis. Since Dr. Hammond first described this interesting member of the family of choreoid spasms, I have seen two cases in which the athetoic spasms were simulated in hysteric women. One of these I saw but once, as it did not return to my clinic; the other was a private patient, and was long under observation.

L. C., æt. 25, from Canada, a stout ruddy unmarried woman, was probably overworked at puberty in acquiring accomplishments which she can no longer use. At 14 she had diphtheria, but no sequent palsy. The hysterical aspects of her case are represented by tendency to tears, by rare hystero-epilepsy, by fits of hysteric coma, by great nervousness, distress at loud sounds and bright lights, and by general abdominal tenderness. Over and above these it is to be remarked that she has a certain general feebleness, not at all suggested by her look of health, nor is she ever very steady in her motions, and is liable to a fine tremor, which subsides only after she has been for some time at perfect rest. Also there is a slight but distinct and very slow oscillation of her eyes, so that this group of symptoms suggests sclerosis. Otherwise she is well, and it may suffice to say so without going into negative details as to sensation, motion, reflexes, and the functions in general.

Possibly this is an hysterical woman with an organic malady, but to which cause shall we refer the athetoic spasms, which I shall now describe? When for relief the hands lie closely locked on her lap, save for a fine tremor little movement is to be seen, but when released, and especially during excitement or attention to them, both hands, the left being the worse, exhibit the most singular motions. The fingers extended, or in extension and flexed on the palm, move to and fro, coming together or separating, or crossing the line of the thumb. These motions are slow, and of a perfectly disorderly character, but they never cease except in sleep and during efforts at any manual work, when they are always replaced by the slight tremulousness already alluded to. In Dr. Hammond's cases, at least in the one given as a type, the movements continued during sleep, and also they were powerful, and there was some pain in the limbs concerned, but none of this applied to my patient. The motions could be easily controlled by another's hand, the resistance being but slight, while also there was no pain. When, however, my patient grew excited or emotional, the movements became rapid, and during her menstrual periods, which were natural, this was also the case. There was no spasm in the feet. The history of these movements is that they arose out of a succession of hystero-epileptic fits, with intervals of stupor, or of stupor with rigidity. At the close of these attacks, although she was in other respects well, the fingers were noticed to be strangely affected, and the disorder thus begun grew slowly worse.

The only question is as to the origin of these spasms. Is it an athetosis proper, or an hysterical imitation of athetosis, or merely athetosis grown, as one might say, on an hysterical soil, and modified by its place of growth? Despite the fact that the athetosis arose directly out of hysterical disorder, I incline to the latter view, especially as in many particulars the case otherwise conforms sufficiently to Dr. Hammond's admirable account. I ought to add, however, that in cases more clearly and purely hysterical, athetoic movements are sometimes met with

In my second case, that of an unmarried woman Miss J., æt. 40, there were slight mental disorder, sensory delusions, left hemianæsthesia, an hysterical temperament, and slight ovarian tenderness (left). Rapid relief of the mental trouble was obtained under treatment, with slow improvement and final cure of the anæsthesia, large gain in flesh and blood, and entire recovery from the hysterical symptoms in general. During the early months of the case there were at intervals attacks of athetoic spasms. Usually these came and went without appreciable cause. At other times emotion, especially terror from her sensory dreams, seemed able to occasion them. They lasted from five minutes to hours, were not violent, conformed absolutely to the type cases, were bilateral, but ceased in sleep, existed only in the hands, and several times ceased when Miss J. was exposed to some diverting cause.

The character of these motions differed somewhat from the utter irregularity of Hammond's disease. I should say they differed unless her attention was called to them, in which case no semblance of order in the spasms could be seen. When unwatched by the patient, the motions consisted in constant slight to and fro and lateral movements of all the fingers, but at brief intervals. A larger range of motion would affect first the thumb, and then in turn all of the fingers in succession from the forefinger to the little finger.

As this woman improved in general condition the finger spasms slowly passed away, and have now, I believe, been absent for at least a year. Whatever doubt there may be as to the hysterical origin of the former case, none can exist as to the last one, so that we may, I think, rank hysterical athetosis among the forms of clonic spasms seen in this peculiar disorder.

LECTURE VI.

TREMOR—CHRONIC SPASMS.

In accordance with the plan I have followed here of treating at one time of groups of symptoms, at another of single symptoms, I shall ask your attention to some of the minor forms of motor disorder found among nervous or hysterical women.

The subjects I shall choose are Tremor, or tremulousness, and certain Spasms, usually local, which are not within the range of hystero-epileptic states, but coexist with perfect consciousness.

You have seen here over and over the tremor of tobacco, of stimulus, of lead, of old age, and also the forms of tremor which are yet more active, such as are met with in shaking palsy and sclerosis. Besides being thus an expression of weakness, as in old age, or fatigue, or the feebleness of convalescence, or of organic disease, or toxic states, tremor is a sign in many people of transient emotion, of fear, of excitement, of anger, or of grief, almost as natural a motor expression in some mobile natures as the facial feature spasm, laughter or crying, is of uncontrolled mirth or grief. Tremor like these, too, is capable, under certain circumstances, of passing over the line of healthy functional manifestation and becoming a symptom of disorder and lack of emotional control. Here we are to consider it as a symptom found often among the nervous, a symptom which may be local or general, temporary or enduring, and may, in a few cases, be so much the most prominent feature of a case as almost in itself to constitute a disorder deserving of being itself labelled as a disease.

If the organic tremors, the offspring for the most part of coarse textural changes, be clearly spinal, it is interesting to ask if the representative tremor of hysteria be in like manner of functional spinal birth, a question more easy to ask than to answer; but seeing the volitional control which many nervous patients possess, as regards the symptom tremor, it seems probable that, in extreme cases, the cerebral ganglia lose those inhibitory qualities which are usually active in the healthy. That, however, this symptom may be of mere emotional origin, or derived from pathological changes, becomes important in diagnosis where it sometimes chances that a spinal malady is painted on a background of hysteria, or that hysterical additions arise in emotional patients to disturb our belief that we have had to do with a malady purely organic. These mixtures of symptoms are, as you will readily admit, when you have seen many such cases, as bewildering as charades. Some of you may recall the case of Miss M., aged 25, a fat and ruddy person, who suffered first from overstudy, combined with some mental worry. At the age of fourteen she had diphtheria, but no sequent paralysis, and came to me a few years ago, at this clinic, a person looking as little like having organic disease as any you are apt to see. About three years before I saw her she had

had an unfortunate love affair, which had ended in a
high degree of general nervousness, a form of trouble
which we have very frequently had occasion to bring
before you, and the symptoms of which, I trust, are now
familiar to you.   It came on rather abruptly, as these
things sometimes do, resulting in a tendency to tremor, which was excited by the slightest emotion, or
the least excitement or worry, and was always worse
at the time of her periods.   We have also interca-
lated, in her case, a brief history of occasional hysterical spasm, with spinal and ovarian tenderness.   It
seems probable that on top of this came a condition
of organic disease of the spine, which is not as yet
fully developed, but which will in all probability end
in a general sclerosis, of the character which we call
disseminated.   She has now some slight difficulty in
walking, vague pains through the limbs, some numbness of the feet and hands, and slight difficulty of
speech, a certain drawling, prolongation of her words,
quite characteristic of the condition in question ; she
has, too, occasional vertigo, and the disk of her left
eye is, I think, suspiciously white, while I find, upon
careful examination, that the vision of that eye is not
nearly so good as on the other side.   The peripheral
appreciation of colors is distinctly impaired, so that
there seems to be only too much reason to fear that
the optic nerves are suffering from atrophic change.
The tremor she has at present may have been originally, and probably was, purely hysterical, since it
came and went, and was more or less within control
of the will.   It has now all the characteristics of a
tremor from organic cause.   She cannot thread a

needle at all, or eat easily, or carry a full glass to the mouth without violent agitation; while the hands are for the most part quiet when at rest. Looking at the whole of the pecularities of this case, it seems to me extremely probable that it has passed quietly, and without the suspicion of her physician, into a state of organic disease of the spine.

You are of course aware that there are two forms of tremor in connection with spinal troubles; I may coarsely state their peculiarities as follows : One is constant while the limb is at rest, and is lessened by motion; and the other is less when the limb is at rest, and is made very much worse by voluntary motion. The tremor of nervousness, and that which is seen in hysteria, may be always constant except in sleep, or may come and go irregularly, without apparent cause, but will always be liable, like some of the spinal tremors, to remarkable increase under excitement or expectation, or the sense of being watched. It is usually a tremor of variable extent, so to speak, the range of disturbance, what I may call the width, being greater than that of most organic tremors, at least at their beginning, while under the influence of emotion, or without known cause, it may pass into a condition of local or general convulsions, the range of motion increasing like the lengthening oscillations of a pendulum. In one respect, however, it distinctly differs from the tremors of organic origin, which are never notably controllable by the will; whereas, in people merely nervous, or hysterically nervous, it is nearly always possible greatly to limit, and sometimes for a time to altogether efface the tremor by a sturdy effort

10

on the part of the patient. The form of tremor of
which I am now speaking, may be confined to one
limb, or may be so general, that almost every part of
the body may be agitated by it, and in these latter
cases, if the muscles of the face suffer also, they are
apt to exhibit larger movements, rather than the finer
tremors which affect the limbs. I remember only too
well the case of a lady, from one of our neighboring
counties, which baffled us completely, a year or two
ago in this hospital. She was a woman, aged 32, thin,
not anæmic, in fact, rather ruddy. The disease began about four years before she came to me, and was a
general nervousness and neurasthenia, caused by a
long spell of nursing two of her family through fatal
maladies. At the close of this effort, which is always
one of the greatest strains that can be put upon a
woman, she broke down with hyperæsthetic conditions
of the senses, with tender spine, with great fatigue on
the least exertion, and with a general failure of her
nutritive functions. I do not remember when the
tremor began, which was so marked a feature of her
case, but I think it was a year from the time of
the first outbreak of her symptoms. When alone in
her room, and thinking herself unobserved, she was
usually quiet, except for a twitching movement of the
face, but when anybody entered and especially when
I myself approached she was seized at once with a universal tremor and with extreme general nervousness,
so that speech became inhibited, and deglutition was
palsied for a time.

For some months, at least, the movements were of
this character, and only after a time grew, what I may

call larger. This was also the history of each onset
of shaking. The motion rose from tremulousness
through large tremor visible to the eye everywhere,
into a tremor which had in it a certain character of
violence, and was varied with occasional slight jerks
of the limbs, and accompanied with perpetual agitation of every muscle of the face, so that she presented
an appearance not less singular than distressing.
This may pass as a good case, in fact, as a rather
remarkable case of general tremor, but you will
understand that this symptom in less marked degree
is very often to be found as an expression of all nervousness, and even of weakness as in convalescence
or in old age, while but few old hysterical cases
escape without more or less exhibition of it.

Localized tremors, I mean such as are absolutely
confined to one part, are somewhat more rare, nor do
I remember to have had the opportunity of exhibit-
ing to you here a single illustration of this class. I
have now under my care, however, a very interesting
woman, who has in both limbs below the knee a condition of tremor, which is about as fair an example of
what I mean as anything that I have recently seen.
In her it was caused by a long strain of nursing followed
by a disastrous railway accident, in which though she
herself was not injured, one of her parents was killed.
It was her general condition for which she came to me,
and the tremor is to be regarded as only one symptom. I was told that some time ago, she was the sub-
jcet of general tremor. She seems to have now a condition of mind not very rare among highly nervous
women, and which without much straining of language

I might effectually describe as mental tremor. A moment of mental indecision seems to trouble her in regard to everything upon which decision is necessary, she revokes her opinion, again decides, and so, but with far more uncertainty of mind than is shown in her speech, comes at last to a conclusion. Her general condition is exasperated by hysterical anorexia, by some dysphagia, and by perpetual and distressing tendencies to micturition, and by violent flushing of the face. Under the influence of tonies, and careful treatment, she utterly failed to improve, but since I have placed her alone, in the care of a a nurse before unknown to her, and steadily fed her every two hours, with also the daily use of massage, she has so rapidly improved, that now there remains very little of these conditions excepting the tremor of which I have spoken, but not fully described. While her hands are perfectly steady her feet are most of the time, or were most of the time, in a state of tremor caused by incessant minute activity on the part of the flexors and extensors of the feet, while there is also a good deal of trembling of the leg and thigh. It has lessened from above downwards. However quiet her limbs, my visit is sure to set them going. She has been taught since she came here to restrain these movements by act of will, at first for a minute, and now for an hour at a time. Aided by the gain in general health, this training of the will has proved efficient, and there is at present hardly any tremor in the right leg, while that of the left is fast disappearing. A well-applied bandage in some way helps her, perhaps as she says by keeping her so reminded of the limb as to be able to dominate it.

A year has elapsed since I wrote the last sentence, and she is now entirely well.

What else need be said of nervous or hysterical trembling has been already spoken of in connection with my remarks on the subject of general nervousness, to which it is so apt to be related. What I most desire here is that you should never confuse it, as you may easily do, with other tremors, but I must have said enough to warn you on that subject.

Alcoholic tremors can only concern us in their diagnostic relationships, and it will suffice if I say, that as to this tremulousness, or other neural symptoms, you should be constantly alive to the rare, the very rare possibility that your patient may owe some of them to the secret abuse of stimulants. I sav the rare possibility, because in a long and large practice among women of the best social class, and the one presumed by some people to be prone to this vice, I have seen but five or six cases of alcoholic drunkenness. I well recall a sad case which was brought to me some hundred miles on a couch, on account of a shocking state of universal tremor, with attacks of prolonged stupor and rarer hystero-epileptic attacks. The woman had been "diagnosed at," as she told me, by many doctors, and took a malicious pleasure in showing me a number of opinions. The tremor was incessant and large, but did not become worse for my visit, although it was at times, I thought, purposely exaggerated, the patient being distinctly pleased at the importance of the role

she was playing. I confess, that I too should have been
deceived as to this case, had it not been for a practice
which you will do well to acquire, a practice now
become with me a deeply confirmed and increasingly
active habit of noticing in a room, not only the patient
but everything else. Missing a bottle of cologne from
its usual place, where I was apt to make use at
times of its contents, I said, "Where is your cologne?"
"My maid upset it," she answered; " she upset it on
the table yesterday; she is very awkward, and did
the same thing last week." My eyes naturally
turned to the table, which was of antique mahogany,
varnished. Now, I had observed that when cologne
falls on varnish it permanently whitens it, but this
table was clean of spots. I repeated my question, and
when the same positive answer came, I was suddenly
sure that she was drinking cologne, and this proved
to be the case. We wrung from her and her maid a
sad tale of the fraud and stratagems by which she had
been able to indulge in this singular habit undetected
for years.

Chronic spasms persistent through months, or even
through years of waking life, are rare enough among
women, but exceptionally rare among even the most
nervous men. The only cases I recall in these arose
from nerve-wounds. In my book on Injuries to
Nerves I quoted but one case, which I had myself
seen. I saw others which had suffered from violent
spasm as an immediate consequence of a ball-wound,
and where, however, the spasm lasted but a few
hours; but was in one case so great that the nails of
the spastically shut hand cut the palm deeply.

You see, therefore, how uncommon is the condition of true chronic spasm, and why, therefore, it possesses so much interest.

The chronic spasms of women with hysteria are, perhaps, among the most obstinately unmanageable of all the graver symptoms of this disorder. They are said at times, by the books, to make sudden recoveries. My own experience as to this is the same as in hystero-palsies. I do not see abrupt recoveries—why, I cannot say—perhaps because the cases which reach me are always old ones, much treated. At all events, you must have seen enough here to know that we earn our triumphs, as a rule, by intelligent and patient care.

These chronic spasms may affect almost any part. You are apt to see the jaw locked; I have seen it kept rigidly open. I have seen the head bent on to the breast, and so held for months. The false tumors of the belly are local spasms of muscles; such a case I saw last year, with Dr. Sinkler, who must well remember how the immense tremulousness told us both what was the constitutional cause of trouble before the woman could uncover her supposed tumor.

Sometimes you will see these very local contractions in a part of other muscles. I once saw two good large, permanent tumors in the calf of the leg. They were merely contractions of muscle, and not of the whole, but of a part, and, like some of the abdominal contractions, were very tender. They came very near to being removed by a surgeon—who, too often, made his diagnosis with the knife.

I have, however, made mention of some of these

cases in a former lecture, and need not dwell here on this especial form of the trouble in question.

Permanent spasms, then, may affect almost any muscle of the body, and be so violent and lasting as to excite our amazement that, through many years, in some cases, a few groups of ganglionic cells should be competent to evolve such enormous amounts of force. I recall from my notes one case, which was, I think, a very interesting illustration of these affections, and which is also worth mentioning to you, on account of the success of the treatment, and because of the various therapeutical experiments, for experiments they must largely be in the treatment of this disease, which were made by others or by myself. This young lady, Miss C., from Maryland, was brought to me a few years ago, as some of my assistants may remember, with violent spasm of all the anterior muscles of the right thigh and leg, the foot, however, being extended. The rigidity of the limb was something extraordinary, it stood out, when erect, at absolutely a right angle to the body, and no pressure that I dared to use was competent to depress it notably without causing extreme pain, and soreness of the stretched muscles. When the hand was placed upon the anterior muscles of the thigh they could be felt to be in a state of tremor, as though not all of the muscular fibres were acting at once. Probably, owing to the long-continued action of the muscles, the limb was never entirely relaxed in sleep, nor during the many months she was at the hospital was it ever seen to be in any other position than at a right angle, or at an angle of 45° with the line of the erect body. A multitude of therapeutic experiments ending always in failure, and the abandonment of the case had been made by several physicians; nevertheless, I undertook the treatment with a certain amount of hope, such, in fact, as I always have, when an hysterical case is taken away from her own home and social surroundings, and subjected to new and revolutionary influences.

I began the study of her case by placing her seated at the foot of the bed propped up with pillows, and then suspended from her ankle an increasing amount of weight, to learn whether I could by degrees depress the limb, and thus wear out the muscles. I have, however, seen her carry a weight of fifty pounds for three hours, and she was but a frail girl, without the limb falling more than a few inches. Under ether the limb relaxed, but there always remained a certain amount of rigidity, owing, I presume, to what I may call the setting of the too long-contracted muscle.

Long before the ether left her, the spasm returned, and, therefore, I was quite sure that it was not one of those forms of mimic spasms of which I have presented to you some curious examples. I next made an effort to wear out the spasm by the use of induction currents, using two batteries, but although I employed such a power of the batteries as could not readily be sustained by any but an hysterical woman, I did not succeed in my efforts, and she remained much as before. The use of galvanism to the spine, no matter what might be the direction of the current, also failed. She was finally cured by very much gentler treatment, which consisted in the use, twice a day, of the fullest hypodermic injections of atropia she could bear thrown directly into the rigid muscles. As soon as the atropia began to show its power in a certain amount of relaxation of the limb, I also had the limb manipulated, having it moved in different directions, upwards, downwards, and sideways. Under this treatment she steadily improved, and finally left the hospital able to walk on crutches, with the limb nearly straight under her, but still unable to employ it in walking. By this time she had obtained a certain amount of volitional control over its action, and in a few months became entirely well. There are cases, however, in which steady extension of the flexed limb, or steady flexion of the extended limb by apparatus will succeed in overcoming this rigidity. Of this I have seen an excellent example in the case of Miss W., also from Maryland, who came to me with the diagnosis of general sclerosis, but who really presented one of the most extraordinary illustrations of hysterical symptoms which I have met with in years. She had at one and the same time some general palsy, a profound loss of power of the left leg, anæsthesia, and chronic hysterical spasm of the right leg, with violent alternate spasms and extensions of the head, together with a quite marked amount of mental hebetude, somewhat rare in such forms of hysteria. To make her case still more difficult, I may add, that she was fat and rosy, in perfect condition, menstruating with ease and regularity, and apparently suffering from no organic trouble whatsoever. I say to add to the difficulty, because I always feel more hopeful of a case of hysteria when it occurs in the person of a woman lean, wasted, and anæmic. You have then, of course, the chance when building

up a constitution, to aid your moral treatment by all
of the profound alterations which you may bring
about during the process of fattening, and filling with
good blood an exhausted system.   In her case I succeeded in extending the limb by the use of a screw
apparatus, and a stirrup fastened to the extended foot,
and attached to the apparatus below the knee.   Perhaps the anæsthesia of the limb may have aided me
in this matter, but, as I have said above, it is not often
that you succeed by these means, and in using them
you may expose your patient to a second disorder in
the form of general convulsions, or local spasms in
parts remote from that first affected.

I saw an example of this in the case of a lady whom
I went to Massachusetts to see, some years ago, and
who suffered from atrocious chronic spasm of the left
arm, so that it was always painfully flexed.   There
was no anæsthesia of the limb, and every effort to
make it straight gave rise, if persisted in, to general
convulsions, which finally caused, as you may imagine,
the total cessation of all efforts in that direction.

The treatment of these forms of spasm must con-
sist in the treatment of the general condition, and of
what that is, I have already fully spoken, in speaking
of the general subject of the course of hysteria.

I have seen tendons cut for these cases, an operation to which surgeons are rather too prone in my
opinion.   I cannot remember a case which was relieved by such an operation, while the use of atropia
hypodermically, and of the slower but gentler method
of manipulation, and in a few cases of extension by
instruments, will in a certain number, assuredly not

in all, bring about a permanent cure. Spasms such
as these, are not often mimicked, but occasionally
you will meet with an illustration in this form of
that unconscious simulation of disease, if I may be
allowed such a phrase, of which I have already so
frequently spoken. In this, and in the mimicked palsies which are yet more rare, there occasionally arises
the chance for those abrupt impressions upon a patient
which so amaze alike the sufferer and her friends.
I recollect, as an illustration, the example of a very
charming young girl from Rhode Island. When I
first saw her she was lying on the bed, with her
knees drawn up, her feet not extended as is usual, but
flexed. I was told that when she awoke in the morning, they were straight, but were almost immediately
drawn up into the state in which I saw them. After
going over her whole system and not discovering evidences of organic disease, I finally made up my mind
that it was a case for one of those bold experiments
which sometimes succeed when more timid action
fails. After inducing her mother to leave the room,
I suddenly straightened one of her legs. I met with
no difficulty until I had partially attained my object, and this proved to me with certainty, that it
was a willed spasm with which we had to deal, and
not one controllable by volition. I then said to her,
" I have straightened one of your limbs, straighten
the other for me." She said, " I cannot, but perhaps
you can." I straightened it with but little difficulty.
I then said, "Sit up on the side of the bed." She replied
that she had not sat up for years, but I finally got
her seated with much trouble, and then, picking up a

gay cravat, and tying it around her neck, I said, laughing, "Now you are all dressed for a walk, how amusing it would be to meet your mother at the door." To
my surprise she yielded, seeming to enter into the fun of
the idea, and with a staggering gait (such as you would
expect from one long confined to bed) she advanced
with me to the door, where she met her astonished
parent who was just coming into the room. She
never went back to bed again permanently, and in a
few weeks afterwards was able to ride on horseback.

You now and then meet with cases in which the
whole range of hysterical phenomena leap into mischievous life owing to some most trivial wound or
other hurt, but it also chances at times that a real
and grave injury of a nerve may give you an
almost indistinguishable mixture of nutritive and
other disorders the usual result of nerve wounds, and
also of hysteric symptoms such as may perfectly well
arise without traumatic cause. It becomes then almost impossible to say of a given symptom, such as
chronic spasm, which may be the child of either parent,
whether it be hysteric or due to the nerve lesion, and
yet as concerns treatment, it may be of the utmost
moment to reach such a decision. The following case
is a remarkable illustration of my meaning.

I saw last year, with Dr. Morton, P. L., æt. 26, a
maid-servant, who had, a year ago, a fall in which
she bruised her left side. Being of a nervous and
impressible nature, it was not surprising that she
was seized at once with left unilateral numbness
and slight loss of power. These symptoms faded
away in a few days as one of the minor injuries due

11

to her fall rose into mischievous prominence. In falling, she struck her left elbow so as to cause pain down the arm, but not in the ultimate distribution of the ulnar nerve. Five days after the accident the pain grew worse, and a general hyperæsthesia spread over the ulnar side and middle of the arm. At the same time the fingers began to flex more and more, until at last all the finger-tips and the thumb came into contact in the position assumed when with all of the fingers we hold some small object. The hand was held in extreme and constant flexion chiefly by spasm of the palmaris longus, the tendon of which was rigid and prominent. The least effort at passive motion of the parts caused intense pain, and the hyperæsthesia was so great that a touch on any part of the fingers, except the thumb and forefinger, and on nearly the whole forearm seemed to occasion the utmost distress.

This case, I confess, somewhat puzzled me. Nerve wounds of themselves give rise in either sex to hysterical states, so that, except for my knowledge of the previous temperament, this condition was of little diagnostic aid. The hyperæsthesia was extreme. It is so in many nerve wounds or contusions, but, at least early in the case, it does not pass out of the distribution of the nerve presumably affected. In this case it did not seem to have any accurate anatomical site, that is, it was partly in the ulnar, and irregularly there, and in a portion of the median and musculo-spiral territories; while there was none of the tactile loss which inevitably accompanies nerve lesions, there being agonizing pain, and yet lack of accurate sense of touch. Besides this, in the present case, the fingers were cold; there were no joint lesions, nor any caus-algia or nutritive changes in the skin or nails. When, too, I pressed on an indifferent point—such as the olecranon process—and led her to believe that I was compressing a nerve, she described her increase of pain as terrible. Either, then, this was a case of slight nervous lesion exasperated by the hysterical tempera-ment, or else it was not a nerve hurt of any gravity, and all of the symptoms had arisen in consequence of a trivial hurt, just as a pin-prick may be the start-ing-point of the most extreme and enduring hysterical phenomena. It would, I think, be difficult to find a better illustration of the difficulties in reaching a dis-tinct diagnosis in such cases, and yet a diagnosis is here, if in any case, most desirable, because, if the case be purely due to contusion of the ulnar nerve, the question of operative interference is certain to arise should the symptoms continue long. This woman was put under the daily use of galvanism to the arm and hand. Each application was followed by relaxation of the contracted parts and by a lessening of the hyperæsthesia. When the poles were applied without making circuit, the same results followed, and I have now not the faintest doubt that the phenomena were from the beginning to the end of purely hysteri-cal parentage.

There is a form of spasm which is sometimes mis-taken for paralysis, and is to be met with, as far as I know, only among women; that is to say, in a large experience I have never encountered a case among men; it is what I might call spasmodic ptosis. It is to be distinguished from that violent closure of the eye which is found with or without some disorder of the fifth nerve, by the fact that it is simply a quiet shutting of the lid, and a resistance on attempting to lift it up with the fingers, and an absolute incapacity for a time to raise it by the will. If this were a paralytic feebleness, there would, of course, be no difficulty in pushing up the eyelid with the finger, but, as I have just stated, this cannot be done without the exertion of a good deal of force. I fancy that, even among women, this condition is rare, as I do not remember seeing more than three or four instances. I mention them as curiosities and as cases which you may occasionally see. There is also a paralytic ptosis which is common among women, and which I hope you will not confound with the malady with which we are now dealing. The last example I have seen of spastic ptosis was in the person of a lady, who came from the interior of Pennsylvania, and who has since died of cancer of the stomach. She was a person easily tired, emotional, and low-spirited at the same time. She suffered also from nasal catarrh, and had, like most of these cases, no photophobia. During the winter previous to her visit to me she began to have, without known cause, a closure of the lids. They would remain closed for several hours at a time, and then would open with probably as little cause as they closed. I saw her twice before I obtained an opportunity to see this symptom. She then seemed to be unable to raise the eyelid, and I could not lift it without a considerable amount of effort. I treated her for a long time, and in various ways, and she had at different times tried galvanism and electricity and many other forms of treatment. Section of the supraorbital nerve had been proposed to her by an enterprising surgeon, but she got well apparently unaided by physicians, and died, as I have said, four years afterwards of malignant disease. Another case was in a woman of great intelligence and remarkable accomplishments who had, I think, injured her brain by excessive devotion to study. She had no disease of the eye proper, nor any organic malady, nor could I say that she was a notably nervous woman. She had, however, been from childhood a shy person, subject to blush too easily, and at times excessively embarrassed by the presence of strangers. The trouble of her eyes came on for the first time at a watering-place. When going to dinner, and sitting down, she observed that a great number of persons were looking at her as a last arrival· she mentioned the fact to her husband, and was almost immediately attacked by a violent closure of the eye, and was obliged to be led in this condition from the table. When this had happened once, you may well imagine that every repetition of the original cause brought back a return of the disorder, until at last it was quite impossible for her to go to table in the room with other people. You will see that in this case emotion, and, after the establishment of the symptom, the despotic control of an unpleasant memory were competent to create and then to continue this grave inconvenience. I succeeded in inducing her, however, to make an effort to go to dinner, without regard to what happened, and

to face the slight unpleasantness and the talk which
her appearance might create.   Her courage was finally rewarded by a cure, which was perfected, so to
speak, by a long absence in Europe, and constant exposure to the very difficulties which had given rise to
her first attacks.

LECTURE VII.

CHOREA OF CHILDHOOD.

SOME years ago I was struck with the rarity of the true chorea of childhood among negroes, of whom a fair proportion applied for aid at my clinic. In the hope of securing more full information as to this question, I asked my friend, the late Professor Henry, of the Smithsonian Institution, to distribute in the Southern States a circular, asking the following questions :—

1. As to the frequency of chorea in white children.
2. As to its relative prevalence in localities.
3. As to its relative frequency in black children of pure breed.
4. As to its frequency in mulattoes.
5. As to the season of greatest frequency of attacks.

This circular was sent, for the most part, to the meteorological and other observers, who were correspondents of the Smithsonian, and through them to their friends. It reached thus a very intelligent class, and fell into the hands of secretaries of State and county medical societies, who were at much pains to give me the collective experience of large numbers of practitioners.

Had all, or nearly all, of my circulars been answered, I could have quite fairly mapped out the relative prevalency of chorea as to States. As it was, my replies gave me the experience of two hundred and ten physicians scattered through the towns and rural districts of the South and Southwest. The information thus obtained is very interesting, and, however incomplete it may be, is too curious to be laid aside. In the hope, therefore, that it may awaken ampler and more exact research, I have ventured to analyze it. No one can feel more fully than I how much it lacks of being perfect as evidence, or how largely it is open to criticism on account of the fallacies, which are apt to pervade information thus obtained.

The points with which I shall deal will be:—

The relation of the chorea of childhood—

To season and meteorological conditions.

To climate.

To locality, town or country.

To race.

Forms of chorea.

Relation to season.—It became clear, many years ago, to every one who followed my clinics, that as the cold of winter faded away, and the changeful weather of March and April prevailed, cases of chorea became frequent. This continued to be the case until, with the warmer season, the number fell away, remaining then at about the same ratio through the autumn and winter months.

These facts were so striking that at my desire Dr. Gerhard collated all the available cases from the note-books of the Infirmary for Nervous Diseases, in order to arrive at an accurate determination of this point in the natural history of the disease. Soon after, Dr. Mills published a like summary of cases from the clinic books of the University of Pennsylvania; and within a few days Dr. Morris Lewis has kindly brought together all of our own cases which have presented themselves since the date of Dr. Gerhard's paper, with additions from my private note-books. This experience thus covers all classes of society.

Dr. Gerhard found that my clinic and note-books of private cases gave for the time of attacks of sixty-eight cases of chorea, thirty-nine in the spring months, ten in the summer, seven in the autumn, and twelve in the winter. This result was sufficiently striking, but was incomplete, because the months of attacks were not indicated. The subject seemed to me to promise interest enough to repay a more exact study, and for this purpose an effort has been made to relate the attack to months instead of seasons, and to examine into the conditions of weather which are to be found in periods of the greatest and least frequency of chorea. For the intelligent study here made of this difficult subject I am largely indebted to the skilful industry of Dr. Morris J. Lewis.

A few years ago no such study would have been possible, but, the resources of the Weather Bureau having been put at my disposal, I have found no obstacle, save in the changes of the method of notation in its tables which have been made from time to time.

EXPLANATION OF TABLE I.

Line 1.   Interpreted by using column of figures 0 to 80; is
intended to represent the *mean relative humidity*, i. e.,
the *mean per cent.*, and not the *mean actual amount*, of
the moisture which could be held ın solution at the *mean
temperature* of each month; the amount representing complete saturation being indicated as 100,—the mean for the
month being obtained from the daily mean relative humidity.

Line 2.   Interpreted by using the column of figures 29.70 to
30.30; is intended to represent the *mean barometric readings* for each month.

Line 3.   Interpreted by using the column of figures 0 to 80; is
intended to represent the *mean thermometric readings* for
each month.   (Fahrenheit scale.)

Line 4.   Interpreted by using the column of figures 0 to 80; is
intended to represent the *actual rainfall or melted snow* in
inches for each month.

Line 5.   Interpreted by using column of figures 0 to 80; is
intended to represent the *months of onset of* 170 *separate
attacks of chorea.*

Line 6.   Interpreted by using column of figures 10 to 20; is
intended to represent the *mean daily range of temperature* for each month.   This is obtained by subtracting the
mean of the minimum temperatures, of each month, from
the mean of the maximum temperatures of the same, and
ıs an ındication of the variableness of the different months.

EXPLANATION OF TABLE II.

This table is merely a mean of the five years 1876–80, and is
interpreted in the same manner as Table I.

EXPLANATION OF TABLE III.

Line 1.   Is intended to represent the *actual* number of days on which *rain* or *snow* fell in the different months of the years 1876–80.

Line 2.   Is intended to represent the actual number of *cloudy* days during the same period,—the cloudy days being determined by the following rule : "In determining whether a day is clear, fair, or cloudy, its character will be determined by taking the sum of the entire number of fourths of clouds, observed at 7 A. M., 2 P. M., and 9 P. M.   A *clear* day will be one in which the sum of observed fourths is 3, or less than 3 ; a *fair* day, one in which the sum is from 4 to 8 inclusive ; and a *cloudy* day, one in which the sum is from 9 to 12 inclusive."

Line 3.   As in Table II. ; is intended to represent the *months of onset of 170 separate attacks of chorea.*

EXPLANATION OF TABLE IV.

Line 1.   Is intended to represent the *number of storm centres passing within 750 miles of Philadelphia* during the years 1878–80.

Line 2.   Is intended to represent the *number of storm centres passing within 400 miles of Philadelphia* (1878–80).

Line 3.   Is intended to represent the *months of onset of 87 separate attacks of chorea* (1878–80).

Remarks and conclusions.—In drawing conclusions from these tables, it must be remembered that, while the meteorological portion is complete as far as carried out, the number of attacks of chorea represented is by no means the complete number occurring in Philadelphia during the five years under consideration, but is merely a list of as many separate attacks as could be collected, where the month and year of onset were known without doubt.

In glancing at Table II. it is seen that the chorea line (5) suddenly rises to a very high point in March, this month having 35 attacks, or 20.58 per cent. of the whole number; the line then falls suddenly in April, then rises slightly during the summer, to fall again and reach its minimum in October, viz.: 6 attacks, or 3.52 per cent.; after this a very slight rise occurs. In comparing this line with the line of mean temperature alone (line 3) nothing especial is seen, the same temperature in the autumn, as in the spring, not being accompanied by an increase of the disease · nor is much light thrown on the subject in comparing it with either the line of the mean relative humidity (line 1), or with that of the mean barometer (line 2), except that there appears to be an increase of chorea with a fall in the mean relative humidity and barometric tracings, and *vice versa*. This can also be seen in Table I., but not as plainly as in Table II.

It has been stated that the disease is most prevalent during moist, cold weather; but this assertion does not appear to be sustained by Table II., where it is seen by comparing the lines 1 and 3 that January, February, and December have a much lower mean temperature, and a much higher mean relative humidity than March, and yet these months have but a small proportion of attacks.

Nothing of any apparent importance can be gleaned by comparing the mean daily range of temperature (line 6) with the chorea line.

In comparing the amount of rainfall and melted snow per month (line 4, Table II.), with the chorea line, there appears to be a slight coincidence, the lines rising and falling together except in May and June, although the amount of rainfall is not proportionate to the number of attacks. In looking at Table III., it is seen that the line representing the actual number of cloudy days (line 2) bears a much closer resemblance to the chorea line than does that of the actual amount of rain and snow (line 4, Table II.). In July and August there appears to be a discrepancy between the two, but in other respects the resemblance is marked; the maximum attacks of chorea, occurring in March, coinciding exactly with the greatest number of cloudy days, and the minimum, in October, coinciding with the minimum number of the latter. The increase in the number of cloudy days in November does not have a proportionate number of attacks of chorea, although a slight rise is perceptible.

Allowance must be made here for the method of computing the cloudy days, as the rule previously stated is not without its objections; for by this it may rain, or there may be a thunderstorm on a *clear* or *fair* day. The line representing the number of days upon which rain or snow fell (line 1, Table III.) also resem-

12

bles, in some respects, the chorea line. This point will be referred to further on, after a study of Table IV.

Line 1 of this table represents the number of storm centres that have passed within a circle, whose radius is 750 miles, drawn round Philadelphia as a centre, during 1878–80, inclusive. The two previous years were omitted, as the storm records were not available. It was originally intended to construct a table showing the number of storm centres that passed within circles of varying radii; but as it was seen that the resemblance between the storm and chorea lines increased as the circles increased in size until the largest with 750 miles radius was reached, it was concluded to simplify the table by only tracing the lines that represent the number of storm centres passing within the circles of 750 and 400 miles radii respectively; the latter line (2, Table IV.) being inserted to corroborate the statement just made.

The reason of the resemblances between some of the lines in Tables II. and III. now becomes more apparent, as they may be considered as component parts of a storm, or as some of the factors of a storm, so that a partial resemblance between them might reasonably be expected. A conclusion which it seems justifiable to draw from the foregoing study is, that no single factor of a storm explains satisfactorily the rise and fall of the chorea line, but it is where these are taken collectively, as in the storm line, that the greatest resemblance is seen.

It is worthy of note here that the chorea line of Table IV. resembles, in all its important features, the chorea line of Table III., although there are 83 fewer attacks included in it, so that it is reasonable to suppose, if a larger number of attacks could be collected, the resulting line would resemblé those depicted in the tables.

It appears that the area over which a storm has its influence is strikingly alike in chorea and in neuralgia, as proved by my former studies in the case of Captain Catlin.[1]

It will be seen with what extreme caution we have ventured to draw conclusions from the elaborate study here made. It is at all events valuable as a step in a good direction.

The facts which come out here so clearly as to the time of choreal attacks and their relation to storm states would seem to indicate the further need for a yet more refined and careful study of other points. It were most desirable in future to set apart the cases of chorea from fright and to study alone those cases in which rheumatism accompanied or preceded this disease, while it would be also most interesting to learn how far the curve of acute inflammatory rheumatism would compare with that of choreal frequency.

It is of course probable that other factors than conditions of weather may have a share in multiplying attacks. One of these is certainly the influence of mental labor. I know of many cases which get well when they cease to study, and relapse at every new effort to do school work. With us the public schools have their most important examination in June, when promotions are made and class rank deter-

---

[1] Am. Journ. Med. Sci., April, 1877. Relation of Pain to Weather.

mined. The pressure on the children is often considerable, and may have its share in the rise of the
chorea line in early summer.

It is interesting, as we pass from this subject, to
pause a moment in order to contrast with chorea, another neural malady as regards their meteorological
factors.

Some time ago my colleague, Dr. Wharton Sinkler,
showed that the paralysis of childhood is most common in hot weather. He has now, at my request,
made out the curves of relative monthly frequency
of this disease as seen at our clinics since 1872, and
has added the curve of temperature. (See Table V.)

The gradual rise to a maximum in August suggests
disastrous preparation by the weather of July, our
month of greatest heat; and the minimum reached in
winter is certainly a fact which no previous theory of
this disease could have prepared us to suspect or an-
ticipate.

Recurrence of Chorea.—The tendency of chorea to
recur is mentioned by several authors, and especially
by Sée. He speaks in one case of six, and in another
of seven returns; and, what is most interesting, he
fixes on the autumn as the time of relapses, as well
as of the initial outbreaks, and thinks that each suc-
cessive attack is apt to be lighter than the last, which
has certainly not held good in my own experience.
The French authors who mention any time for occurrence or recurrence of this malady all follow Sée's
statement. According to him, the six autumn and
winter months furnish three-fifths of all the choreas.
This he attributes to the joint action of cold and

moisture, which seem to him the most important factors, but which, as our tables show, does certainly not hold good as regards this country and latitude.

Dr. Gerhard's paper mentioned the facts observed in this direction at my clinic, and in my private practice. Out of 80 cases, 25 had been attacked before. Of the 25 cases, 14 had thus had chorea three times; 8 had had it twice; and 3 had experienced it four times. Of the 25, nineteen recurred in the spring.

My later experience has given me cases of chorea which have recurred in a yet more remarkable manner. One young girl had chorea for four years either in March or April; then once in February; and then for two years in May. In another case the disease broke out in a lad æt. twelve, and recurred every spring for three years. In a third case, the disease began in a girl of seven, and missing one year persisted until she was thirteen, when it ceased to appear. The attacks began usually in March or April.

I never knew a case to recur thus pertinaciously in the autumn, although sometimes, in this latitude, vernal attacks get well in summer, and recur in autumn. The same holds good of winter chorea. If cured, there is a positive tendency to break out in the spring.

Dr. Morris J. Lewis's table of my own clinics gives this result as to repetitions of attacks: 126 cases, representing 185 attacks.

Since I have been well aware of these facts, I have been accustomed to warn parents of the tendency of chorea to recur, and have always given careful instruction as to the general treatment of the child in

winter, and have always given arsenic as the spring
began. I have in this way broken up, in many cases,
the habit of vernal recurrence of chorea.

How far such facts hold good of other latitudes than
this I cannot yet say; but I gather from many of the
letters of answer I received from our warmer States,
that the onsets of this disease are probably more common in winter than with us. I have no accurate
numbers wherewith to settle the question. It would
be very interesting to know what law of occurrence
and recurrence chorea follows in Great Britain.

Relations of Chorea to Climate. Locality.—After I
had determined the factor which I have here illustrated, I became somewhat interested in the question
of climate as related to this disease, and was soon
struck with the slight information on this subject to
be found in the books. Von Ziemssen says that
Hirsch has now authoritatively contradicted Rufz's
statement of the rarity of this disease in the warm
zones both in black and white. Its relative frequency
is hard to judge of, because there is little or no death-
rate, and because cases are sometimes noted as deaths
from chorea, when they were due to other maladies.
Hence the only evidence is the statement of physicians in active practice.

If I consider this, I should conclude from the
answers to my questions, that warmth does not numerically lessen it, as in fact my tables show. It
appears to exist in all of the larger cities all over
our Southern States, and also quite freely in Cuba.
Dr. Finley, of Havana, and Drs. Landetta and De Cas-
tro, formerly of that city, report it as common enough,

especially among girls at the approach of puberty. I hear like accounts from Lisbon and from the great cities of South America. In a few cases Southern physicians write me that it is rare even in large towns, but when they add the number of cases they have seen, it is usually clear that they have met with quite as much of this disease as it is common to encounter at the North. The facts already pointed out, which show clearly enough that chorea is seen most in the spring and early summer, might very well prepare us to find least of it in such localities as the Bermudas, where the temperatures vary so little through-out the year; but as to this I have no information.

There is another factor in the case, and an impor-tant one. It comes clearly out in the answers I re-ceived. Chorea is a disorder engendered in some way by the evil influences which are found wherever men live crowded together in masses. It is essentially a disease of cities. The larger cities, both in the north and south, furnish it, as I should judge, in much the same proportion. There is less in the smaller places, and in country practice, north and south, it is an ex-ceptionally rare disease. Physicians who have been twenty to forty years in rural practice, sometimes cannot recall a case, and yet, as we know, rare cases are usually the best remembered. Among one hun-dred letters, were twenty representing—and it is no bad way to put it—over three hundred years of prac-tice by men who have never seen a case of chorea.

I should at least have expected to find, that, in highly malarious countries, where, as we know, the endemic influence tells severely on the health of all ages, this lowering cause would be competent to do what some combination of atmospheric causes enables the spring and summer months to do—awaken chorea. There is, however, no evidence to favor the view that chorea can have a malarial origin, except that it arises in spring with as much certainty as ague. But there is also some direct evidence to show that there may even be something hostile in malaria to chorea—a point which I make with considerable doubt. It would seem, however, that, in localities where malarious plains are bounded by wholesome hills,—as a most excellent observer, Dr. Ellis, of Elkton, declared, and some other physicians also,—the chorea which they met with arose on the hills, and not on the plains. To this I should add, that, in certain of the most malarious regions of the South, chorea is a nearly unknown malady.

It would naturally follow upon what I have said, that the disease itself would be found to increase numerically in cities in direct proportion to their growth. Of the increase of a rarely mortal disorder we can however, have no just conception, and the deaths reported as due to chorea must, as I have said, be regarded with a certain amount of suspicion, and this remark will especially apply to years long past when there was far less accuracy of discrimination as to the causes of death from neural maladies.

The slightest study of the vital statistics of our own cities will show how just is this criticism. In Chicago from 1851 until 1866 there is no report of a death by chorea at any age Then in 1866 there is one, a girl of 15 years, and then none to 1869, where my statistics fail me. The population had meanwhile increased from 38,000 to 252,000.

In Philadelphia, between 1807 and 1881, chorea is given as the cause of death in 64 persons, of whom 38 are said to have been under 20 years, and 26 over that period of life. In this list are many over fifty and many under two years, so that there were probably in these two sets a fair proportion of imperfect diagnoses.

Race.—Although aware of the insufficiency of the material on my hands to answer thoroughly this question, I have felt unwilling not to use the letters which so many gentlemen have been at great pains to write me. I have, however, hesitated the more because the tentative opinion on this question which I reached quite early, has been criticized by very able southern physicians as not in accordance with the facts they themselves had observed.

Let me admit, to begin, that in these letters there may be many errors; that rare cases may be forgotten; that the negro often fails to call on a doctor for even serious maladies; and, granting these sources of distrust of my statistics, I do not see how we can fail to conclude as I have done, not that the negro is insusceptible of having chorea, but that in the black race it is far more rare than in the white.

Of sixty physicians who replied at length—some lived in cities or towns, some in the country—twenty-seven speak of chorea as rare in the white; all of the rest give the number, or an approach to the number, of white cases they can recall. One has seen an epidemic outbreak of chorea. Of these sixty, forty-nine have never seen chorea in the black; the rest who write speak of it as rare, or mention having seen single cases. I should add that many of the examples spoken of were women, but exactly of what ages is rarely stated.

Even this curious correspondence of view does not, however, impress me so much as the character of the writers of some of the letters and the extent of inquiry which they have made. It may be well worth while to analyze portions of this evidence.

Dr. B. De Landetta says, as regards Cuba, and two others indorse his opinion: "I have never seen chorea in the negro, which is strange, because it is rather frequent in Cuba among white girls at puberty, and because rheumatism is common in the negro." Dr. Ch. Finley, of Havana, thinks chorea rare among whites; but, despite his appeal to the Havanese Academy of Medicine and the publication of the questions in its journal, but one case of chorea in the black could be heard of.

Among the letters are several from physicians who had been large owners of slaves, and had also had extensive plantation practice. One, Dr. Ashe, of Alabama, having seen in all seven white cases, never saw a case in the negro.

Dr. Benj. Lee writes that in a year of service in the Hospital of the Home for Colored Children, New York, he saw a case of chorea in a mulatto girl æt. 15 end fatally, but has never seen it in the pure black. Dr. Kollock writes me from Cheraw, S. C., that he has seen in twenty five years of large practice some twelve cases in the white and two in the negro of pure breed. Three physicians write me from Louis-burg, N. C., that one of them in thirty-six years of practice recalls six or seven cases and one death in whites. Two others have seen a few white cases, and none of the three any black cases. Prof. J. L. Cabell recalls but five cases in the white, and has seen none in the black. Prof. Bemiss, of New Orleans, has seen cases both in white and black, and does not feel sure as to this question. Dr. Ellis, of Elkton, Md., a most competent observer, has obtained, by careful inquiry, knowledge of thirty cases in the white in ten years, and of two in black or colored children. Dr. Michel, Montgomery, Ala., writes me that no one of the thirty members of their County Society ever saw a case in the pure negro. The disease is seen in whites. The secretary of the Medical Society of Columbia, S. C., from correspondence in the State and from the debate on this subject in the society, was unable to discover a case of chorea in the negro.

Dr. Peyre Porcher, having put this question to thir-teen members of the Charleston, S. C., Medical Society, received for answer that the disease is not common among whites, and that no one of the number had seen a case in the negro, and to this, Prof. E. Geddings adds testimony to the same effect. Dr. Laurance, of Hot Springs, Ark., says chorea is found very rarely among negroes, more often among mulattoes, but is not a common disease where he has lived in the South. The general evidence in Virginia is very much to this effect, but in Richmond it is clearly less infrequent, both in white and black or colored, than elsewhere in the State.

On the other hand, many physicians in Virginia state that it is as common in one race as in the other, and Dr. Landon Edwards, of Richmond, after a careful inquiry, reached the conclusion that the negro has no immunity

It seems to me, however, that as the matter stands, the weight of evidence is in favor of the opinion that the black is less liable to chorea than is the white.

Varieties of Chorea.—I pointed out some years ago, that there exist at least three groups or species in the genus chorea of childhood. The significance of the distinctions is not as yet clear to me, but I am inclined to think that they may indicate a differentiation in the anatomical sites of the central disturbances which give rise to this disorder. As they are not yet adopted in the books or confirmed bv the researches of others, I shall venture here to restate briefly my views so as sufficiently to illustrate the peculiarities I have seen.

Group First.—The common type; awkwardness and incoördination of voluntary movement, followed soon or late by automatic or unwilled clonic spasms of various parts.

Group Second.—The disease never gets beyond the first stage of incoördination. Just as in some scleroses of the cord there is no tremor save during volitional acts, so here the irregular motions only occur during willed actions.

Group Third is, I think, the most unusual type, but I see occasional cases every spring. In this there are constant automatic, irregular, clonic spasms usually of the hands, but during volitional acts these entirely vanish, and the most complicated acts are well performed and without obvious incoördination. In other cases voluntary motion merely lessens the spasmodic activity, but does not abolish it. It is necessary to illustrate only this third group.

T. C., æt. 14, female, applied at my clinic in May, 1879. She was a florid healthy looking descendant of healthy people, but had one brother who was epileptic. In March, 1878, she was attacked rather suddenly with clonic spasms of both hands. These parts were in incessant movement during the waking hours, and until she attempted some acts of volition. Then, and during the movement in question, they were entirely free from all appearance of incoördination. She could write, sew, lift a glass of water, or do any other act involving complex motion without the least tremor, but in a moment after it was done, the fingers would again resume their spasmodic activity.

I have seen a number of these cases. They are distinctly choreal, and yield to such treatment as is of value in that disease, but they differ plainly enough from the ordinary type of chorea.

13

LECTURE VIII.

HABIT CHOREA.

I HAVE over and over in my clinics called attention to a disorder of childhood which is the source of some anxiety and more annoyance both to parents and physicians. This trouble I venture here to label Habit Chorea, and for reasons which, I think, are good and which will appear in full as we consider the cases.

Over and over some anxious mother will ask you to notice her child on account of some little trick or gesture in which the child indulges. Then you will see that it is winking rapidly, or pursing up the mouth or drawing it to one side, or, perhaps, that the brow is lifted at intervals or a shoulder shrugged, or some forward movement of the jaw or head is repeated over and over at varying intervals.

These acts occur usually in children of either sex, but I think most often in girls from 7 to 14 years of age. In many cases the single grimace or motion is repeated for months and then disappears, and, if this were all, I should hardly think it worth while to label so trivial a disturbance of health; but in other cases the first habit is lost by and by, and another takes its place, so that the variety and obstinacy of the habits become troublesome and even cause alarm; or, worse still, the little patient has a large repertory of these performances, and will execute a remarkable variety in one day. Usually, in such instances, there is some one motion which is more violent or more frequent than the others.

If you examine with care the history of these little patients you often find that there has been some fall from the plane of health, and you will at once wish to know wherein the child's life and work and play are not what they should be. Sometimes finding nothing to blame, you will recall the fact that, in the process of growth, children undergo cyclical changes which are not permanent, and which in turn may bring or take away tendencies to neurosal disorders, so that you must not always expect to be able to detect the causes of such disease.

If you analyze more closely the character of the symptoms we are studying, you will find quite enough to repay attention. You will observe, first, that attention to the child increases the trouble, and that any little failure in health has a like influence. Then, if you see many such cases, you will observe that these children are sometimes irritable or excitable, or exhibit clearly enough a condition of nervousness, being more emotional than is natural; while, in a few instances, they lapse into well-pronounced chorea of the ordinary type. In fact, this disorder has a certain kinship to the latter affection. If you ask an intelligent child, who is thus diseased, why it makes the grimaces, or repeats, at intervals, some odd movement, you will learn that, while the patient is able, in most instances, to restrain itself and control the exhibition of motor disorder, this restraining power becomes increasingly difficult the longer such effort lasts, and that a certain malaise or discomfort results; while to give way and let the morbid impulse have full sway is attended with a sense of comfort and relief.

Such is, in brief, all that I know about this small malady; although you will, perhaps, comprehend it better if I relate cases and point out, by illustrations, the fact that its treatment should be very much that which is needed in full-fledged chorea; another argument, if a slight one, in favor of the relationship of the two disorders.

During the present month of November I saw M. C. G., æt. 13, girl. Never a robust child, at the age of six she became, without known cause, nervous, restless, and irritable; and was, for awhile, a bad and uneasy sleeper. About this time she began to have a slight hacking cough which came and went; was made worse by an attack of scarlet fever, and still exists at times. It sounded like a cough which was forced and voluntary. At nine or ten years, the cough almost passed away, and was succeeded by a sort of snuffling, during which she made the usual grimace, always on the left side, and precisely such a movement as accompanies snuffling. Whenever she makes this contortion she pushes her cheek up with the left hand. For a long while the cough and the snuffling act continued, the one or the other being prominent for a time. She was scolded and bribed into making great efforts to stop these morbid acts, and more or less succeeded. The next summer she was taken to Saratoga, and the cough and snuffles abated, but a new symptom arose. The mouth would be opened wide, and as it closed both eyes shut, and remained closed for a moment, or else this took place without any opening of the mouth.

When I saw the child, all of these odd movements were in full activity, but usually one of the three was more frequent than the others. There was at this time a good deal of dyspepsia, sluggish appetite, and pain in the back low down, probably indicative of the coming on of her menstrual flows, the approach of which was rendered probable by a rapid development of her bust and pelvis. She had had no worms, and no organic or functional disturbances other than those I have mentioned. As she is just now, for the first time, under treatment, I can say nothing as yet of its success. Careful and good diet, light gymnastics, no school, gentle aperients, and full doses of arsenic constitute such therapeutics as seemed to me reasonable. I ought to add, that she does not seem in any degree mortified at her own peculiarities, and this will be met by some effort to make the matter appear to her as rather disgraceful, and not to be mentioned—something, in fact, to be ashamed of. I shall be much surprised if this combination of physical and moral treatment fails us.

The next case I shall relate is quite as good a type. This was a lad, aged fourteen, who was taken from school a few months before on account of twitching and nervousness. He had become also irritable and capricious, and the grimaces, for which chiefly he was brought to me, had increased, and had, indeed, been

increasing from the previous April, and until he gave
up school late in July. It is in fact usually safe in
such cases as this, and in all choreal troubles, to predict either a return or an increase of the symptoms in
the spring.

In this lad the twitches began with snapping of the
eyes, and this came and went, but was never quite
lost, but merely lessened when some new symptom
arose. The second form of trouble consisted in a
curious rolling of the head, difficult to describe. This
was bad enough, but quite suddenly within a few
days the face became more quiet, and there arose a
disorder of the abdominal muscles which were
abruptly contracted at intervals. Over this and over
all of these motions my patient had a good deal of
control. If he set himself to hold it in check, this
was possible so long as he steadily attended to the
task, but while it was easy to repress it for fifteen
minutes it was difficult after half an hour, and increasingly more and more hard, until by and by some
slight lack of attention enabled the act to recur, or
else the sense of discomfort and strain involved in
these resolute acts of will power became unendurable,
and the lad abandoned the effort. After a month or
two of these movements, the respiration was broken
every few minutes by a sudden long drawn abrupt
inspiratory act. Still later the head was affected,
or rather the neck, with a little short negative shake.
The abdominal and respiratory disorder gave way at
last to shrugging of one shoulder, and then to this
with a queer upward pull of the whole side. The
worst attack lasted but a few weeks, and was a sort of

straightening up of the body. These varying conditions endured for several years. At one time the boy seemed well, then spring time or any little malady, especially indigestion, or much study and in-door life seemed to reproduce the troubles in some shape new or old. It was a slight grimace to-day, and in a week or two it was a sudden action of the muscles of the back or a shrug or a spasm of the muscles of the belly. In no case did the hands or feet suffer, and always the disorderly act was distinctly controllable by will; this repression was unpleasant, and some relief was found in allowing the muscles to have their way.

As the patient's eyes were plainly imperfect, Dr. Noyes, of New York, was so kind as to send me a statement to the effect that the lad had, in the right eye a slight mixed astigmatism, and in the left a slight compound hypermetropic astigmatism. These errors were really trifling in amount. The eye muscles showed some weakness. The eye grounds were healthy.

I had a long bout of treatment with this lad, whose docility and good sense lent me every help.

He took at first a good deal of valerianate of zinc, and had cold douches to the spine, and also arsenic internally. Meanwhile he was taken from school and set free in Virginia on the sea-coast to ride, swim, shoot, and fish. Notwithstanding these wholesome aids, we got no further in the way of relief until we began to use hypodermic injections of arsenic. For this Fowler's solution without the lavender was used thrice a week, in doses rising from two drops to twelve, and as this heroic medication was followed by rapid subsidence of the symptoms, it was continued for nearly three months. A sea-voyage and residence at an English school completed his cure, and then we had also the favoring influence of approaching puberty.

These cases, and I might readily add others, sufficiently illustrate the varieties and the peculiarities of the disorder to which, for reasons which must now be plain enough, I have with some hesitation given the name of Habit Chorea. The last case also defines sufficiently well what the treatment ought to be.

LECTURE IX.

DISORDERS OF SLEEP IN NERVOUS OR HYSTERICAL PERSONS.

THE man before us is a feeble anæmic creature, who complains that he has become nervous, an ill sleeper, and has lost weight. · He is a coffin maker, and looks as if he were artistically fitted for some such ghastly labor. He has no organic malady, and I only speak of him at all because one symptom of his case is of sufficient interest to serve as a text.

He tells his story well, perhaps more dramatically than I can, but with less brevity than I need just now. When falling asleep he is conscious of something indefinable, not describable, rising from his feet and going up to the head. Usually he can move and thus check the progress of the disorder; sometimes he cannot and then the attack results in a sense of something like a blow struck on his head. At first it created terror, now he has become used to it, and is no longer alarmed, although the expectation of it is unpleasant, and apt to keep him awake.

This is a mild form of a very curious symptom—I can hardly call it more—which is quite common among hysterical women, more rare among men, and which exists in a variety of forms, and is in such persons at times a difficult symptom to deal with, and in certain cases the parent of a great deal of mischief. In 1875, I published a brief paper[1] on some of the disorders of sleep, in which I described these phenomena as follows :—

'The trouble I shall describe is rarely found alone, but makes a part of one of those groups of neurosal symptoms which have no place in the books, and which are apt to vary largely.

'M. A., a prominent physician from the Northern States, after a season of greatly excessive labor, became rapidly anæmic and weak, and developed the following symptoms: tingling, numbness, and heat of the extremities—now here, now there—on the chest, face, or scalp. At times, after much fatigue, islands of vasal paresis, seen as slightly raised purple blotches on the feet, are observed, and frequent waking up at night, with numbness of either arm; feeble sleep, a dull, occipital pain, which made him wish to hold the part; singing in the head, referred now to the occiput, now to the ears, but an inconstant symptom. He was at last driven to consult me by the following symptoms, which caused him the utmost alarm.

'When just falling asleep, he became conscious of something like an aura passing up from his feet. When it reached his head, he felt what he described as an explosion. It was so violent and so loud, that for a time, he could not satisfy himself that he was not hurt. The sensation was that of a pistol shot, or as of a bursting of something, followed by a momentary sense of deadly fear. This sense of an aura is, as Brown-Séquard wisely says, not confined to epilepsy.'

[1] Virginia Med. Monthly, Feb. 1876.

I have now in my care, a very accomplished gentleman, whose case is in almost every respect like that just sketched, except that the numbness is never universal. The victim (Mr. V.) is, in this instance, a slight sensitive scholar, not overworked, but too steadily worked, which may amount to the same thing. In him, the numbness of the finger-ends came on abruptly, but as in the other case, there is no true loss of tactile sense, and possibly, nay probably, the feeling belongs to some condition of the lesser blood-vessels of the part, and only secondarily to the nerves.

He feels, as he is falling asleep, a sense of something about to happen, but no distinct ascending aura. If he arouses himself in time, for which at the moment he clearly comprehends the need, he can by turning over relieve himself and break the chain of morbid events. He can even watch, as it were, the coming of the shock, and in some way know the moment beyond which he must not wait. The first patient described as suffering in like fashion has also remarked on this peculiarity. Mr. V. has rarely the sense of a pistol-shot or a blow on the head. "I have," he says, "at the close of the attack, a noise in my head, which is sometimes like the sound of a bell, which has been struck once, and I have in my case listened as to a bell, to the vibration coming and going at rhythmical intervals, or else I hear a loud noise, which is most like that of a guitar string, rudely struck, and which breaks with a twang." The result is always, however, a sense of dread, but not such a death terror as has Mr. A.

I have been told by other persons, that they were

liable, when going to sleep, to have sudden sounds, faint usually, and rarely loud, but without feeling of terror.

Since writing this account I have seen a large number of persons who suffer in like fashion from some one of the various forms. The most of the cases are women worn out, or tired out, and hysterical, whether strong and well nourished or not. In sturdy men it is rare, unless they be excessive users of tobacco.

The disorder in question I never saw in a man, except in the border land between waking and sleeping. He may have the aura and then the subjective sensory phenomenon, or the latter may come without warning; but in hysteric females these attacks may arise either at the moment of going to sleep, or during the day at any time, and while fully awake. At times they are slow in the march of their symptoms, and may be checked by the patient if, what is rare, she have enough of resolution; but very often the aura rises fast, too fast to allow of action or of emotion, or else just slowly enough to give time for a sense of fear, the full development of which requires a certain amount of time.

The warning by an aura is common in women thus attacked, and consists either in an indefinite sense of something rising towards the brain from the feet or hands, or both, or else it is a distinct tingling.

In a smaller number of cases the only warning is an impending sensation of pure terror, which increases until the sensory shock occurs. But as regards all forms of the aura, or warning sensation, it is found that, as a rule, the intensity of the emotion weakens with repetition.

The aura is totally lost in the phenomena which follow. These may be classified as follows:—

1. In the sphere of general sensation: sense of a blow, of shock on or in the head, of rending or bursting.

2. In the auditory sphere: loud noise like an explosion.

3. In the visual sphere: flash of light.

4. In the olfactory sphere: sense of odor.

5. A combination of two or more of these sensory manifestations.

6. More or less abrupt and general motion, the ordinary outcome of any violent and sudden sensation.

It will repay us to analyze somewhat more minutely the pecularities of these interesting attacks, since I have usually found that they are not only sources of alarm to patients, but of doubt and puzzle to their medical attendants.

In the first group the final symptom is referred to the head, and is a feeling of a blow, violent or light, struck on the skull; or it is a feeling so terrible as to be described as something like an explosion, or a pistol shot, or more vaguely as a shock, something undefinable and terrifying.

The auditory forms are described in their varieties as a noise, an explosion, the sound of a bell, a booming sound—that of a guitar-string rudely struck.

The visual form is simply a flash of light, with or without sense of noise.

14

The single case of an olfactory form of sensation will be more fully described hereafter.

The affections of general sensation may exist with auditory symptoms or not, since, when it is possible to get a patient to evolve, out of the terror and confusion of such attacks, an analysis, they usually mention some disturbance of audition as going with the sense of a blow.

In rare cases the patient is left with a momentary vertigo; more often the start which announces the sensory symptom ends the attack, so far as its immediate phenomena are concerned. Not so, however, its results in the emotional sphere. In some persons it gives rise to great alarm, even after many repetitions of attacks, and in these and others is apt to leave the victim shaken and hysterical, or to be the first of a series of hysterical symptoms, the end or exact future of which no man can predict.

I would like now to illustrate some of these interesting symptoms by cases, always asking you to remember that in this lesson, as in some others, I am picking out a single symptom for study, and that it is not always the main feature of the case.

The following case is told so well in the language of the sufferer that I prefer to leave her account almost unaltered. It is one of a few rare examples in which the shocks occurred at times while awake as well as during the state of sleep. A series of severe mental and physical strains, and a slight sunstroke left my patient, a woman, now over fifty, anæmic and reduced to the weight of seventy-six pounds, her height being five feet three inches. Her eyes and ears were healthy, her womb normal. There was no trouble of any internal organ, but there was a loud soft hæmic murmur at the right side of the base of the heart. Her sleep was good as a rule, but was easily disturbed and insecure. She writes thus: "Some years ago, when thirty-nine years old, after a long bout at nursing, sustained by quinine and stimulants, I began to fail in health, and then first became subject, whether asleep or awake, to a sensation, which I can only describe as a wave going through my head and threatening as it seemed to me an unconsciousness which never came. If in bed, I would start up, and if riding or walking would clutch at some near object for fear of falling, yet I cannot remember to have felt unstable. The following summer, after slight heat-stroke, and a new exposure to severe fatigue of body and mind, I experienced, once only, a sensation like the explosion of a pistol in my head. I hardly know how otherwise to describe it. A few months later, I began to have what I have always since called my shocks. A peculiar something, which for want of a better name I call electricity, starts from my head, chest, stomach, or bowels, and seems to pervade me in a flash, then comes the sense of shock in the head and an uncontrollable shriek. At first, it never came unless my eyes were shut, but for one week when I was most highly nervous and sleepless, it would come if I was startled by any sudden sound, and then I found that for a short period I could cause it by touching a spot over my stomach.

"Of late, these shocks are not always preceded by any length of warning, and are in the head alone.

They come mostly as I am going to sleep, and by straining my eyes to keep them open, I can some-times prevent the shocks altogether. I should say, that there is often some queer sense of chilliness in my head for an hour before the shocks, which is in a general way a warning of what may come. I do not like to so restrain them when the ten-deney is strong, as I then have one or two during the night while asleep, when they are very frightful to me. In some cases there will be a succession of weak shocks, and at last a strong one, when I shriek. After absence from home and freedom from cares, I have been exempt from these shocks for weeks or months."

This unhappy case I mention first, because of its obstinacy. I have rarely seen the shocks thus per-sistent, and I am sure that they will disappear when-ever this woman becomes vigorous. Neither is the case quite typical, like one I have lately seen, and which readily got well. It is valuable because the shocks were so much the most prominent symptom.

Early this winter, Mrs. L., of Massachusetts, æt. 45, a ruddy, hale looking woman, five feet four, weight 156 pounds, came to me with this simple story: She was well until her husband met a year ago with disasters in business. Her anxiety about him, and the worry attendant upon the management of a household with suddenly lessened means, were made worse by the grave illness of her only child. She became nervous under these influences, and began to suffer from sounds which commonly cause no annoyance. Then her sleep got to be imperfect, and she had a series of hysterical attacks—the usual spasms—trismus, rigidity, hysteric coma, and the like, with a slight but distinct and general lessening of acuity of the sense of pain and of touch. Finally these phenomena passed away, and about this time she became subject to the shocks I have spoken of. These occurred either at the moment of going to sleep, and while quite conscious, or in the day-time, and when wide awake

The aura began in both feet, and ascended rapidly to the head, sometimes being felt also in the hands and arms. It was described as an air, and at times as a faint tingling. It ended in a sudden sense of a loud report, which caused her to seize her head with both hands, and left her in a state of alarm and feebleness, and with a brief but tumultuous throbbing of the heart. The attacks took place irregularly, once a week at first, and later at much longer intervals. Their effect was disastrous, because they gave rise to distressing nervousness, and sometimes to prolonged hysterical conditions, in which all her usual hyperæsthetic states were remarkably accentuated.

While she was under my care I saw a lady from New York who was a sufferer from a variety of nervous symptoms, dependent in part on a split cervix uteri and a lacerated perineum. These were surgically relieved through operative means by Prof. Goodell, but the after-treatment of the hysterical conditions, hyperæsthesia, sleeplessness, and intense general nervousness was a slow process. The use of ether during the operation, which I have learned somewhat to dread in grave hysteria, seemed to be the immediate parent for

14*

a time of an increase in all her old symptoms, and of some new ones, among which were the shocks.

The attacks came at any time except in sleep, and were similar to those of Mrs. L., but less severe. There was no aura, unless we can so call a feeling of impending peril, which lasted a few seconds, and ended in a sensation of a blow on the head. The attacks ceased after a month, and have never returned.

The next case I have to relate was more curious. A girl, æt. 18, was placed in my care some years ago suffering from a slight unilateral hysterical paralysis, with well-marked anæsthesia. She was far less nervous than the woman I have described, and, in fact, it is, I think, not rare to find that women with distinct hystero-palsies are, if we omit ovarian tenderness, fairly free from the various hyperæsthesiæ which constitute one of the groups of hysteric symptoms. She had, however, attacks when going to sleep, in which she became conscious of a something which seemed to ascend from the feet to the head. If she could rouse herself, or turn over, the attack terminated, and usually did not recur that night. It sometimes happened, however, that she was not able to act in time, or was clearly conscious that she could not, in which case there was a wild flash of vivid red light, and she was at once seized with distressing nervousness, and sometimes with tremor. I do not remember that the attacks ever took place when awake, while it is as certain that they never occurred during sleep.

The next illustration of the double sensory discharge giving rise to subjective feelings of sound and light is valuable, because the account is given to me by the sufferer, a medical officer of the United States Army, R. M. O'R., æt. 35, married, parents living, both of gouty diathesis. He is, and always has been, strictly temperate in all respects. Smokes in moderation. When twelve years old, had a sharp attack of intercostal rheumatism. In 1868 contracted malarial fever, from which he has suffered more or less ever since. In 1867 received a trifling gunshot wound of right thigh. In 1875 had concussion of the brain, and some injury to back, resulting from a fall. Was confined to bed for a week or ten days, and walked with difficulty for some time after. Was troubled with vertigo for over a year. Has had no other sicknesses nor injuries.

In June last, while sitting lost consciousness; did not fall. On recovering, saw objects surrounded by a halo; walked home with some difficulty, and went to bed; slept none that night, but occasionally dozed, and was awakened by a sensation of falling, or by a sudden noise, or by voices calling. Remained in this condition for about two days; could arouse himself, but as soon as the effort relaxed, dozed, and had the feelings described. This condition gradually wore off, leaving vertigo, appreciable muscular weakness (especially of the lower extremities), a sense of constriction around the head, wakefulness, and want of appetite.

Late in June came to Philadelphia; consulted Dr. Alison, who observed that one pupil was somewhat dilated. Subsequent ophthalmoscopic examination by Dr. Thomson showed nothing abnormal.

Early in August went to Oswego, and has passed

the time there and thereabout until a week ago.
Within the past month has had two or three severe
headaches, with pain, over the left temple. These have
followed fatigue or excitement.

At present he can walk but a short distance without growing very tired, then comes vertigo, seemingly
confined to the posterior portion of the head, and a
condition of nervous exhaustion, lasting some time.
The same effects ensue upon mental strain of any
kind. He sleeps fairly well. The feeling of constriction around the head is constant. Appetite variable,
but never very good; bowels inclined to be costive;
temper irritable; want of capacity to think a subject
out, or to decide any question; has lost weight. No
organic trouble of heart, lungs, or kidneys.

Since June last he has had several shocks, of an
explosive character, which appeared to be within the
cranium. They came at irregular intervals, and
without assignable cause. They have always occurred
just as he was falling asleep, and have been preceded
by no abnormal sensations. He is awakened by what
seems to be a loud explosion in his head, accompanied
by a flash of white and blinding light. There is no
pain with it, and except an acceleration of the pulse
there are no sequelæ. The noise thus heard is described as a rather low note, accompanied with a feeling as if the head was sundered by the explosion.
The attacks come and go, but are always so dreaded
as to make him dread the going to sleep.

I have notes of a yet more singular case, which I
hesitate a little, and perhaps without due cause, to class
with these.

A woman, æt. 40, and in good health, was hurt during the tumult which followed the explosion of the boiler of a steamboat. She was thrown against the rail of the boat, striking her nose violently, and then fell into the water, whence she was rescued insensible. For several weeks she was very ill, and recovering became the victim of acute hysteria, which in a year passed away, leaving her feeble and emotional. Her sense of smell was entirely lost from the time of her accident, and except that she had at times a subjective and very annoying impression of the presence of an odor of brown soap, she had had absolutely no appreciation of odors.

When I saw her two years after her accident she had, at long intervals, these symptoms. At any time, awake or asleep, she became aware of something like a touch moving over her, usually about the epigastrium. After a few moments she experienced a sense of shock in the head, usually at the back of the head, and with it a remarkably distinct sense of a strong odor, like that of bananas. It persisted for, as she thought, a minute or more, and then slowly faded away.

I have seen a number of these cases of sensory shock, and I suspect that, when inquired into, we shall find them less rare than might be supposed. The instances I have related cover most of the varieties I have seen, and it only remains to say a few words as to their clinical relationships, diagnosis, and treatment.

The clinical relationships of these attacks are to epileptic fits, and to those well-known, and, I may say, normal phenomena of a sudden movement of the body at the moment of going to sleep, or even at other times, to which I shall presently refer again.

The analysis of the shock attacks is simple. The basis is hysterical excitability, or a hyperæsthesia from tobacco, or overwork with worry. The attack itself is preceded in many cases by an aura of some kind, which is the first sensory expression of the coming disturbance. The aura is a phenomenon of general sensation. Then follows a more or less violent discharge from a centre of general sensation, as of a blow or shock; or from auditory centres, a noise as of a bell, a guitar-twang, or an explosion; or from visual centres, a flash of light; or, perhaps, two centres act at once; and there may be no aura, as in many epilepsies.

The fact that these attacks do in some people take place in the waking state, removes them from dream phenomena, and from the domain of nightmares and of night-terrors; one form of which occurs in the interval between sleep and waking, and presents some analogies to these attacks of sense-shock.

In this form of night-terror, which is seen rarely, but has often enough been described to me, the sufferer is perfectly conscious of the coming on of a nameless dread. Something precedes it in the way of a warning. He can, by an act of will, escape it by motion, or he may watch its onset. When it culminates it is merely a state of insensate dread or terror, without a felt cause, dreamed or other. This seems to me, in the mental or mere emotional sphere, to be closely akin to the sensory shocks.

As to diagnosis I do not see how these attacks can

well be confused with anything else, unless with the minor epilepsy, from which it ought to be easily enough distinguished

As to treatment there is not much to say, but what there is to say is important and interesting.

As we are dealing chiefly with the nervous maladies of women, the cases in which sensory shocks are caused by tobacco and excess of brain-work do not so immediately concern us here. I may, however, be permitted to say that in all symptoms directly traceable to tobacco there are two remedies available while the habit is being broken, strychnia and alcoholic stimulus. It should be needless to say that the man who orders the latter ought to have some security that his patient will not construe his orders too liberally. But this is a matter for a doctor's conscience; and, at least, he may feel secure that a little whiskey at bedtime will correct the evil results of over-use of tobacco, and may be left off as soon as the tobacco is much lessened. As to strychnia no warning is needed; and Dr. Landon B. Edwards has pointed out, and with reason, that it is the tonic most useful in the feebleness which comes of abuse of tobacco—that pleasant wife and fatal mistress.

As to cases of sensory shock in women, the real remedy lies in treatment of the conditions out of which it grows. Of these, I have already said enough, but there is one matter as to which, in the nervous maladies of women, it is hardly possible to say enough.

Perhaps I had better introduce what I wish to say in this direction by a brief extract of a letter from a woman who has suffered gravely from the shocks I

have described. She says: " I suffer, as you are well
aware, from these shocks in the time between sleep
and wakefulness, and also in the day-time, though
rarely then. It did not seem to me at first possible
that I could in any way control these attacks or
save myself from their results. I found, however,
that, as I had warning enough, I really could do so.
So I set myself every night to be resolute to turn
over or sit up if I had a warning; and every day I
said to myself, if I have the warning to-day, I will
not yield, but jump up and run about. To my surprise, I found that by following out this determination with resoluteness I could break up most of the
attacks."

The treatment hinted at in this letter from a clever
woman is really valuable. It consists in instructing
the patient before going to sleep, and every day, to
keep in mind the need to break the attack by motion
and by an effort of will.

I do not know of any drug which is directly useful
in such cases of sensory shock as seem too grave to
await in patience the influence of general tonics.
The bromides are, in competent doses—such doses as
make deeper sleep than common—dangerous to nutrition or at least hurtful enough to be avoided if possible; and in the small doses, in which they do good
in hysteria, are, as regards this particular symptom, valueless. Small doses of chloral or morphia,
used until the habit be broken, answer well; but still
better is a general improvement in health, and then,
if the attacks persist, such exercise as will insure
natural fatigue deep enough to make it impossible to
avoid sleep.

In the same paper on sleep to which I have already alluded occurs some brief account of the motor discharges which are so familiar to us all as taking place just at the moment of deepening sleep.

What I pointed out then, and what I wish to recall attention to here, is that this normal symptom, if I may be allowed so to call it, does sometimes rise into the mischievous position of being the dominant difficulty in a case on account of its interference with sleep.

The symptom in question—while it rarely takes place except in the interval between waking and sleep, and never between sleep and waking—may also arise during sleep itself, and cause abrupt disturbance. I have seen it very troublesome in growing lads and in some overworked men; but it is rare to find it so strikingly developed as in the case of a woman who consulted me to-day. This unfortunate person was forty-three, the mother of several children, and of late irregular in her menstruation. I was struck with the fact that her color was good, but that she was curiously thin and very haggard. She is well as to her digestion, but has too much wind, and finds eating hard work; otherwise she is well in the day-time, and can read, sew, walk. or drive, as pleases her. Once or twice she has had long crying spells, without other cause than a sense of the wretchedness of her condition. When bedtime comes she goes with fear and reluctance to encounter sleep and the discomfort it brings to her. Just as she begins to lose herself, an arm, a leg, or the whole body suddenly moves with violence. As she awakens, her

15

hands and feet, or either alone, twitch for a few moments. Then she settles herself to sleep anew, only to repeat the same process, until at last she sits up, crying hysterically, or, worn out, falls into a slumber seemingly too sudden and profound to allow of the phenomena I have described. Her daughter, who came with her, described these nights of suffer ing as truly pitiable, and told me that nothing had as yet seemed to afford the least relief.

Of late, Mrs. R. J. has been apt to wake up later in the night with unilateral tingling, of which I shall presently speak more fully.

You must of course consider this as an unusual case ; but it is just unusual cases which are apt to puzzle young physicians; and to be able in such cases as these to recognize the close kinship between an almost natural phenomenon and its excessive develop- ment into an annoying disorder, is not only comforting to the patient but useful to the physician.

A good many hysterical women exhibit this symp- tom ; and in a few it becomes troublesome, either bv its repetitions, as in Mrs. R.'s case, or, what is less com- mon, from its severity. A quite ludicrous example of the latter I saw a few years ago. The patient was one of those stout, ruddy women, with good ovaries, and uterus where it should be, and yet hysterical to an exasperating degree. She weighed over 200 pounds, and was unhappily subject to what she called "fish- flaps," which were really remarkable, because her body would be thrown up from the bed so high, and descend with such violence owing to her weight, that it was not rare to find the slats of the bed giving way. She grew better as her hysteria lessened, but is, I believe, still subject at times to these unpleasant and undesired gymnastic symptoms.

There is yet another and a very interesting sleep symptom seen at times in Duchenne's disease, and in a variety of degrees in some feeble and anæmic persons; but far more common among women than among men. I ventured some years ago, in speaking of it, to call it "night palsy," or "nocturnal hemiplegia." Since seeing more examples I perceive that brachial monoplegia is its most common expression.

This curious symptom assumes one of two forms— the one common, the other rare. In the more usual cases the sleeper awakens with numbness, or rather tingling and numbness, of one arm, a leg alone, which is infrequent, or the whole side, including the face, and even the tongue, which is now and then attacked alone. The disorder may be mere tingling, or actual loss, or rather lessening of tactile sensation; but in any case it rapidly fades away, or yields to a little friction. At first, while it is in the arm alone, the patient refers it to lying on the part; but this becomes an impossible explanation of the hemiplegic examples.

As I have seen in a month three cases of this rather interesting condition, it cannot be very rare. It is significant, perhaps, that some persons who have gotten pretty well of a hemiplegia of organic cause are liable to awaken out of sleep with numbness and lessened power of the side once palsied. It is remarkable that in the case of Mrs. R. J., of which I just now spoke, this same curious functional hemiplegia would at times occur on the same nights when she suffered from motor discharges.

The less common form of night palsy is, perhaps, also the more serious, but may be like the usual examples, but an expression of hysteria or of the exhaustion felt by an ill-nourished brain during the long fast of the sleeping hours. In it the patient exhibits a far more distinct loss of unilateral power, which, however, lasts for an hour or more after awaking, and may even become worse for a time in place of at once improving.

I recall very well the case of Mrs. C. L., æt. 27, who, after profound blood losses in confinement, nursed, with success, through several excessive menstrual periods. She then had an attack of nocturnal hemiplegia, which became more grave during some hours, and yielded easily to faradic stimulation, iron, and good diet. She had after this several light attacks, and twice well-marked brachial diplegia, which lasted but a few hours. I should add, that there was no renal trouble, and that she made a perfect recovery.

Among other milder forms of trouble, which at times haunt the sleep of nervous or hysterical females, are palpitation of the heart, vertigo, and a certain failure of the respiratory centres, which is met with also in grave shape in some cases of Duchenne's disease, or in any very feeble people, and is, of course, not confined to women.

In locomotor ataxia, towards its paralytic stage, this symptom is but an expression of a defect in the medulla oblongata, and has twice in my knowledge finally resulted in sudden death during sleep. In feeble and hysterical people it means simply a temporary failure of function, owing to imperfect nutrition.

The centre remains competent so long as the will is free, during the waking hours, to assist the automatic activity of the ganglia, but when sleep leaves the regular succession of respiratory acts to the unaided powers of defective nerve-cells, there sometimes comes a moment of temporary incompetence, and the patient wakes up gasping and alarmed.

The best remedy for these troubles is to be found in the general treatment, of which I have already said enough, and in great care to supply nourishment at bedtime, and if needful to repeat its use during the night. Of course I take it for granted that every care shall have been given to the state of the stomach and bowels; and I may add, finally, that some patients suffer less, or not at all, if lying on one side or the other, or on the back, the position of success being purely a matter of experiment.

LECTURE X.

VASO-MOTOR AND RESPIRATORY DISORDERS IN THE NERVOUS OR HYSTERICAL.

I HAVE over and over called attention in my clinics to some of the many and curious vaso-motor disturbances which we see in so great variety among nervous women. From the heart to the capillaries we are liable to meet with conditions of disorder, which are sometimes almost as lasting as if they owed their parentage to obvious and coarse structural lesions. This indeed is a familiar fact which I have had ample opportunity to verify both in my clinic and in my private practice. No matter what be the form of general nervousness or the variety of hysterical illustration, the nervous supply of the heart or vessels, or both, almost never escapes from bearing some part of the mischief, and only too often, after everything else is well and the patient is afoot and able to live as pleases her, she will still be reminded by something in connection with the blood supply and its channels, that they are almost the last to regain the vigor and steadiness of health.

The first point to which I wish to ask your attention is the pulse. In the mass of hysterical women, and especially in those we see here who are apt to be feeble, and easily tired as well as liable to tears and to more distinct expressions of the hysteric temperament, the pulse is apt to be permanently rapid, that is for months or years it mav remain 20, 30, 50 pulsations to the minute above the normal number. You may see this in a woman who is supine in bed, and who for the time presents no startling evidence of general disorder. I shall have presently to illustrate this fact by cases.

But besides the speed of the heart movement these cases present also two other phenomena; their hearts are irritable and prone to beat rapidly owing to causes which are powerless to affect the less excitable organ of the healthy. Then also with this cause of being set going beyond their common rate these hearts are apt to become irregular, and to seem to tumble about in an alarming manner. The careful study of these well-known peculiarities will very well repay us. Therefore, before going further we will linger a little upon the questions connected with the pulse rate and rhythm of nervous or hysteric women.

Out of half a dozen good cases I take two or three to enable me to illustrate these points. After that I shall point out some of the eccentric pulse symptoms, and then say a few words as to the mode of dealing with the irritable heart of the nervous, either when it is but a symptom, or when it rises into such prominence as to be the dominant mischief.

There was last year in the Infirmary for Nervous Diseases, a lady from Virginia, who presented in a typical form the cardiac states which I expect to find in neurasthenic women, and especially in such as are both feeble and hysterical. She was 38 years old, married but childless, and had been for some years subject to hysterical attacks, which passing away left her at last so feeble that she was unable to walk up stairs without great exhaustion. She was five feet one, weighed one hundred pounds, and was anæmic and sallow. Her uterine functions were fairly good, and she suffered no pain and had no distinct uterine disease although both ovarian regions were tender, and pressure upon them caused nausea and vertigo, as well as other phenomena to which I shall presently refer. Her digestion was good if she ate but little at a time and was not tired or excited.

Her heart when she was lying down was never under 130 beats per minute. Any exertion raised it 20 to 30 pulsations. The least excitement did the same, but despite this irritability the rhythm was always good, and I should add there was no affection of the eyes or the thyroid gland. Pressure on the ovarian region gave rise to sudden increase in the number of heart beats, but pressure on the spine almost anywhere had a like influence. She had tried absolute rest for a week or two at a time, and had taken a large amount of tonics and of digitalis. Her temperature was curious, being in the mornings 97–97.5°, and in the late evening, 9 to 10 P.M., 100–101.5°, although there was no pulmonary or other visceral trouble. The evening pulse was usually a few beats under that of the morning.

Electricity (induced current, slow interruptions) used as a muscular exerciser, and also massage, excited her greatly, causing tremor, tearfulness, and a rapid increase in the pulse. Withal, the heart was perfectly healthy as to its valves and its size.

I began her treatment by using various forms of digitalis, but although she took enormous doses I never succeeded in making any impression on the heart and usually this drug seriously disturbed digestion. I found that frequent small feeding with rest somewhat aided her, but although she was thus made more comfortable there was no substantial gain, until in despair I resorted to Carell's skimmed-milk treatment. After three weeks of this I was able to repeat the use of massage which I had been forced to abandon. From this time the improvement in flesh, color, and self-control was notable. When she was able to walk about after two months of rest, the heart had fallen to 95° and was far less excitable, and her temperature had become normal. It required, however, many months of care to make her circulation quite natural, but within six months she became fat (one hundred and thirty pounds), and was able to complete her cure by a summer in the mountains.

This was, of course, an extreme case of cardiac nervousness, but it is no unfair type, and I need add little to the description. Sometimes the tumultuous action of the hysterical heart is the most distressing and most upsetting of all the many symptoms of this disorder, so very fertile in symptoms. We all know how unpleasant and appalling even is the sense of sudden and great irregular palpitation, and in the nervous and hysteric this impression loses nothing of its terror. You will meet with such women—women whose hearts seem to become wildly irregular on the least provocation, or on none. Digestion in these women causes it, and here I cannot too earnestly insist that digestion, like some other functional acts, gives rise to symptoms which are not of necessity proofs that the function in question is imperfect or diseased. Ordinarily, if we have palpitation of a healthy heart during digestion, that means often enough that our patient is dyspeptic, but not so in nervous and hysterical women. Digestion naturally quickens the pulse, and in these people the normal quickening passes into palpitation. That I am correct as to this is shown in the same women more rarely by the varied disturbances which follow the most perfect performance of other normal functional acts as simple as micturition or defecation. I have seen patients in whom bowel movement always produced irregular heart action, and I have now a lady under my care who has, soon after passing water, slight chilliness, twitching of the face, and extreme palpitation of the heart. Yet, the act of urination is, in this case, painless, and, in fact, absolutely natural. You may regard all of this as of trifling moment, but I have seen cases like these treated with many drugs, and in a case similar to the last one I have known a surgeon resort to dilatation of the urethra. Bear in mind, therefore, that sometimes in nervous people the activity of a normal function is competent to cause distress or awaken symptoms.

The violence and singularity of the pulse-signs in true hysteria are beyond expression strange.

I saw, very many years ago, a handsome girl, of twenty, from Cincinnati, who had spells of apparent

death, if I may use such a term. One of these I had
the good fortune to see, and indeed to cause, for hav
ing been warned by no one that, to speak before her
of certain things, was apt to cause the trouble, I
unluckily began to discuss with her the subject of a
personal peculiarity, from which I had been told she
suffered.

It seemed that certain odors would, in her, bring
on hysterical attacks. You may recall a case here,
last week, of an aphonic girl, in whom musk would
do this. Now my patient had, at last, become very
sensitive as to this as to other matters, and no one
near her ventured to talk about odors; since then it
seemed that the young lady was liable to suffer, as if
from the odors themselves. Of late the hystero-epilepsy had given place to the "Death spells," as her
friends called them, and it was one of these I pro-
voked. She said to me, "I am going to have an
attack; feel my pulse. In a few minutes I shall be
dead." Her pulse, which just before was about 100,
was now racing, and quite countless; while the
irregularity and violence of the heart's action seemed
to me inconceivable. With the interest of an hysterical woman in her own performances, she said to
me, "Now watch it; you will be amazed." This certainly was the case. Within a few minutes the pulse
began to fall in number, and, as well as I can recall
it, in some fifteen minutes was beating only 40. Then
a beat would drop out here and there; the pulse
meanwhile growing feebler, until at last I could neither feel it, nor yet hear the heart. In this state of
seeming death, white, still, without breathing or per-

ceptible circulation, this girl lay for from two to four days. In this time there were spells of a few minutes, during which the heart beat again furiously and irregularly, as was also the case when she revived.

Of course, emotion of any kind is, in such women, able to disturb the heart-rhythm and its number· and while such persons are subjected to the contacts of daily life, it is, therefore, hard to relieve them.

The oddities of hysterical cases are perceptible enough in the way in which the heart-action seems, at times, to disobey all apparent laws, and baffle all predictive skill. I have seen such persons, whose hearts beat slower when they rose, and faster when they were lying down. I have now a patient, whose heart is quiet enough while she is supine, but to lie on either side causes palpitation and increased rapidity of pulse.

There are now in the Infirmary two cases of great general nervousness with hysterical histories. Neither has organic disease. The one has an average morning pulse of 100, and a night pulse of 75. The other nearly reverses these numbers, but I have been utterly unable to find a precise cause for these peculiarities.

Apart from cardiac troubles, or in relation with them, are certain vaso-motor disturbances which give rise to very distressing, or, at least, to annoying troubles in this class of sufferers.

Every hysterical woman is liable to a certain want of tone in the surface-vessels which gives rise to a group of disorders, owing to which we meet with extreme states of pallor or of flushing which in some cases affect the extremities and in others are most visible in the face. This want of steadiness in the vessels of the skin belongs to some extent, and naturally, to others than the class I speak of, and is seen very well in certain healthy women of fair complexion, and is also common in persons who are liable to the congestive type of neuralgic headaches. Watch one of these women, and, if they have this peculiarity in a high degree, it will come out under the excitement and embarrassment of clinical questioning. You will then see the face flush, and the flush by degrees break up into spots of red which move slowly and have bounding margins of paleness; and all this will be best seen on the neck and cheeks and below the ears. At the same time the hands and feet may become cold, and, at all events, you will find that almost incurably cold feet are the constant annoyance of these patients; and sometimes the cold feet are pale; and sometimes, in graver hysterical cases with palsy or sensory defects, they may be purplish; and both appearances indicate, as you know, defects of blood-supply, and both lead to like results.

Another and very remarkable indication of the acquired sensitiveness of the surface-vessels in cases of the hemiplegia of hysteria is the well-known fact that any moderate traumatic injury to the skin-vessels gives rise to their instant contraction, so that slight wounds which usually bleed do not do so in them. I have seen this state of things in hysterical girls who were not suffering from analgesia, but in most cases it is found over a half of the body affected by some loss or lack

16

of feeling of some kind. As the feeling improves, the
needle wound bleeds, and whatever aids the one condition helps the other, so that, when from the use of
metals the phenomenon of transferrence of the anæsthesia to the opposite limb occurs, it is at once found
that needle wounds cease to bleed on the side attacked
and bleed on that deserted by the disease. As I said
in a former lecture, I have myself been unfortunate
in never yet having been able to see the phenomenon
of transfer. I have several times seen metals laid on
the anæsthetic parts give rise to some partial return
of feeling and of bleeding from needle-pricks, but I
have seen caoutchouc and wood and even sponge do
the same; and the effect of a blister and of the rhigolene spray can be seen in a patient now in the wards.
I may add that dry cups and mustard have also given
me the same results. There may be indeed some
unsuspected relation between loss of sensation and the
bloodlessness of slight wounds, for in one, at least, of
those remarkable cases of total surface anæsthesia to
all forms of sensory impression, in a case of profound
melancholia, although the loss of feeling extended to
the face and mouth, and was certainly not hysterical,
the surface was made to bleed with the most extreme
difficulty. The same phenomenon of failure of pin
pricks to bleed has been recently observed by me in
a man with hemi-anæsthesia of cerebral and organic
cause. It seems likely that cutaneous ischæmia is to
be added to the list of symptoms which Charcot has
pointed out as common to hysteric hemi-palsies, with
loss of pain-sense, and the hemi-anæsthesia of more
definite cause. Since I was led to suspect that there

is some link of relation between anæsthesia and surface failure to bleed, I have been on the lookout for a case of nerve section in which to test the matter. Two days ago, Dr. R. J. Levis cut the sciatic and crural nerves in a man who has a deep and incurable ulcer of the left leg. This operation deprived him of all sense below the middle calf, and I was enabled, with Dr. Levis's permission, to examine the case in his ward at the Pennsylvania Hospital.

All forms of sensation were extinct in the foot. Using a very large needle, I left it in place some time, or turned it about freely, but was unable to cause a single drop of blood to flow from these repeated wounds. As I withdrew the needle, a small, snow-white ring, slightly raised, formed around the orifice, and seemed to be due to contraction of the neighboring skin muscles. This most interesting observation confirmed for me what already I had seen some years ago in other and less extensive nerve sections. I had, however, continued to doubt the correctness of the former observations, which were made in cases of division of ulnar or median trunks. It certainly seems as though the loss or lessening of sensation were associated with the taking off from the skin vessels of some inhibitory influence, so as to leave them to contract with violence under the influence of any irritating cause. All explanations may admit of question, but as to the fact to be explained, I think there can be no further doubt. I hope that I have here said enough to direct attention anew to this interesting phenomenon.

Temporary flushing or pallor of face is very apt to

accompany sudden and irregular heart action, and to become and remain a distressing symptom. Why, with a perturbed heart, this woman should have a deadly paleness, and that a profound flush of face, I cannot say, but both sets of conditions are familiar to me. Now, as in such females the heart becomes agitated, and the face red or white on the least provocation, or on the mere expectation of it, you can readily see what an annoyance it may become.

I saw last year a bright, intelligent New England girl, who, with much general nervousness, had also a heart far too rapid, but besides its speed, if she met a friend suddenly, or went into a drawing room, or was even spoken to unexpectedly, her heart became irregular, and her face very pale. You may readily imagine to how much misconception such a disorder might give rise. The longer it lasted the worse it became, and one pleasure or one duty after another was given up in turn, because of the shame to which every mildest emotion subjected her. After long treatment she became well as to most of her ailments, but had been a year in seeming health before her circulation re-acquired the proper tone, and she could again face, without fear, all the trials of social life.

Flushing with tumultuous heart action is more common, and is, I should say, more like an exaggeration of a common functional event of health. Still, when it occurs habitually on the least emotion, it is, like any such symptom, a source of most bitter annoyance.

Unilateral, or strictly local flushing, is, I suspect, a very rare affection, either in hysteria or elsewhere, but, of course, the best examples are to be found in hysteria.

Last year I was consulted by a lady, both of whose legs were as red as blood in excess could make them, and this state came on after many months of varied hysteric troubles. Excepting an imperfect paraplegia these had all passed away for the most part, but whenever she sat up, her legs filled with blood and looked as if they might burst. Unlike cases of erythromelalgia there was no pain, and when the limbs were elevated they slowly got back their color. Pin pricks bled easily, and there was no loss of feeling. I watched this singular condition for some weeks, every effort failing to relieve it, and finally, I may add, when it was let alone, and only the constitutional state was looked after, the local paralysis of vessels gradually got well.   •

I have over and over seen this vasal paresis in the hands of these women, and one distressing case of intense and permanent redness of the face, which took at first a unilateral form, and then attacked the entire face in spells. These began at any time, but chiefly in the morning hours. A spot of color came anywhere on the face, went and came, and at last others appeared. These coalesced after a time, and the color darkening the face, scalp, ears, and upper neck seemed like those of a heavy drinker. There was no pain, or only a sense of uncomfortable fulness and heat. The eye-ground did not seem to share so fully in the vascular fulness, but the depths of the ears did. Relief was obtained by a spray of cool water, which did best at a temperature of 50° to 60° F. If let alone

the redness passed away slowly within three hours.
At first, and at times afterwards, the heart's action
was disturbed a little.   I should add that very prolonged use of digitaline seemed, with care of the
general health, to do the most towards the complete
relief of this unhappy patient.

The last case of hysterical vaso-motor manifestations which I shall quote was so amazing that if I had
not had the good fortune to see it over and over, and
to show it once to my friend Dr. William V. Keating,
I might reasonably have hesitated to tax the credu-
lity of my hearers.

Some twenty years ago I attended a young married
woman, whose life was embittered by losses of property, and by the ill-treatment of her husband, who
finally deserted her.   For a long period she exhibited
at times hysteric disorders in the forms of spasms,
rigors, hemi-palsies, and at last for a month or two
moderate maniacal excitement.   With favoring circumstances she at last got well, and removing to the
west, was lost sight of until about ten years ago,
when I was called to see her at a hotel in Philadelphia.   At this time my patient was 35 years old,
was irregular as to her monthly flow, and had, as I
found, a womb tilted forward but not diseased, and no
ovarian tenderness, or at least no tenderness of belly
which was not the same everywhere.   She was rather
pale, and very thin, and had a relaxed pendent belly
marked by the scars of four pregnancies.   I could
find no disease of heart, lungs, or kidney.   She gave
me this brief history: After some years of ease and
comfort, she had been led to risk her property in

a wild speculation which ruined her, and now she was keeping a boarding house in New York, and was doing well, or likely to do well, except for the strange malady on account of which she came to consult me. After her new misfortunes she had some hysterical troubles, but these ceased to annoy her, and she began to observe that at or about the time of her menstrual flow, and afterwards at any time, she was liable to have an enlargement of the belly, which did not seem to her to be due to wind, as with that form of swelling her previous experience had made her but too fully acquainted. The trouble became by degrees worse, and at last was so extreme as to cause certain unpleasant feelings, and to subject her to suspicions of being pregnant.

The swelling was certainly caused at times by emotion. It began at any time, rarely at night. Within a few hours the belly, in place of being flaccid and pendent, was swollen enormously. She looked, in fact, as a woman, thin as she was, would have looked at the eighth month of pregnancy. Other attacks were less severe, but always they lasted for some hours before she could stand up, and it was usually a week before she was well

When I saw her an attack was at its worst. The woman's pulse was about 165, and was a mere thread at times imperceptible. Her face and limbs were white and cold. The abdomen was tense and red, and could be felt to throb distinctly, while all over it the vessels, veins, and arteries were visibly enlarged. On listening over the belly I could hear a humming noise, a slight thrill. The chest itself was not quite

so pale as the neck or face, but the breath was difficult and rapid. It was clear that owing to palsy of
all the abdominal vessels, all the available blood of
the body of a too bloodless woman was for a time in
this cavity and its walls. If while in this state she
sat up she instantly fainted, and it was difficult even
to lift her head, because of the symptoms thus caused.
She herself complained of the tension of the belly,
and of the distressing pulsation within it.

The day after the abdomen was certainly a third
less, and it was then seen by Dr. Keating, who, like
myself, could give no other explanation of the condition seen, than the one I have just mentioned.
After a week the belly became nearly as flat as usual,
and I then ceased to see my patient. I learned from
her some years later that by slow degrees she had
become well of this singular malady.

Yet a few words before I abandon this subject as
to the irregularities of breathing in the hysterical.
These may accompany cardiac disturbances, which
is rare, or may exist alone, without elevation or
altered rhythm of pulse. In other forms of disease,
as you well know, when the breathing becomes rapid,
the pulse also proportionally increases in number;
and it is uncommon to see excitement of heart from
fever or inflammation without a like rise in the rate
of respiration; but hysteria breaks all laws, except its
own rules of eccentricity.

I have seen a woman with a respiratory rate of
10, and a pulse of 100; another, with a pulse of 30,
and a normal speed of breathing.

There is now in this hospital a case of hemi-anæsthesia and hemiplegia, getting well after two years in bed. When she began to walk about, two months ago, her pulse was 60 to 70; her respiration 15 to 18. My assistant soon after observed that the rate of breathing was increasing, and, without calling attention to it, we began to keep daily notes of it, and of the heart and temperature.

The average pulse, early in November, was 75–85 in the morning and evening respectively. Respiration 16–17.

At the close of December the pulse had slowly risen to an average, for the two daily observations, of 94.1, with, nearly always, a rather faster pulse in the mornings; but, meanwhile, the breathing rose to a daily average of 49.4.

Some of the numbers are remarkable. I give in a brief column one week, for comparison with healthy states :—

	Pulse. Morning. 10 A.M.	Respiration. Morning. 10 A.M.	Pulse. Evening. 10 P.M.	Respiration. Evening. 10 P.M.
Dec. 22.	102	50	91	48
" 23.	100	52	99	53
" 24.	98	57	100	62
" 25.	90	55	87	47
" 26.	95	37	85	39
" 27.	98	55	88	44
" 28.	93	49	88	89
Mean	99.3	50.7	91.1	47.2

The respiration was singularly tranquil, despite its rapidity, and there was not the slightest appearance of effort. Digitalis, given in half-ounces of the infusion, seemed to have no effect on the pulse after some

days, but so disturbed the stomach that I was forced
to give it up. The thirtieth of a grain of sulphate of
morphia brought down the breathing one-fourth, and
the one-twentieth of a grain had a still more perceptible effect, so that the average fell for the last week to
28.1, while the pulse held an average of 81.2. A
single full dose of opium, given to relieve pain,
brought the respiratory rate from 58 to 17 within
a few hours; the pulse falling at the same time from
88 to 73.

This is a remarkable example of a rather unusual,
but sometimes overlooked hysterical symptom. In
a doubtful case it alone would decide the diagnosis;
for a like condition, outside of hysteria, is a clinical
curiosity. The most remarkable illustration, not hysterical, is that reported by Dr. J. H. Brinton and myself. A man, after receiving a ball through his right
lung, continued for years to breathe at the rate of 100
to 130 to the minute; his pulse being 85 to 90.

I said that this abnormal rate might alone decide
your belief in its hysterical cause; nor is this a
mere theoretical idea. A few years ago I was one
of three physicians called to see a lady, long ill with
a variety of ailments. She had passed into a state of
stupor, from which, for two days, it had been impossible to arouse her. I observed that while her pulse
was about 90, her breathing was almost imperceptible; on careful count, however, it proved to be 96 in
the minute, from which I was sure that the case would
prove, in the end, to be hysterical; an opinion justified within a few hours by the repeated occurrence of
very violent hystero-epilepsy.

LECTURE XI.

HYSTERICAL APHONIA.

THE patient before us to-day is a very notable illustration of the pranks which may be played by hysteria. I read you her history, and as you hear it I think you will see that almost at any time a resolute man, whom she trusted and who understood her disorder, could have saved her and her family from long years of suffering. Her case will enable me to point out to you, as I have done very often before, that the natural history of many of the forms of hysteria is still an open study. One reason for that is I presume the disgust with which the general practitioner encounters this malady. It is hysteria, and with that seems to end all need for observation of details and varieties of symptoms, such as more manageable disorders obtain.

Mrs. R., æt. 31, from New Jersey, was brought up among people of narrow means and larger wants. A rather frail constitution and nervous parents doubly prepared her for the ills which were, perhaps. only hastened by an attack of ague, followed by pneumonia, in September, 1870. Soon after recovery a day of fatigue and some worries ended in hysterics, with retention of urine. A more violent fit followed an attempt to do some rather hard work. From this time the Pandora's box of hysteric ills was opened, and they came almost without limit. Remaining in bed, fit followed fit, until, when a little better, she chanced to smell musk, upon which she fell into a state of stupor, and was thought to be dying. Then the voice fell to a whisper, and so came and went for five years, and at last failed so utterly that for the last five years she has uttered no sound. Meanwhile she stayed in bed till 1872, and had, in succession, general paresis, right arm and hand paralyzed, enormous swelling of hand so as to resemble an abscess, and a variety of hyperæsthesias; on one occasion a blow on the hand caused retraction of the head, followed abruptly by recovery of previously lost power. Soon afterwards there were in succession repeated attacks of hemiplegia, renewed hysterics, paralysis of left leg, and swelling of foot, with exquisite hyperæsthesia of the whole skin. In September, 1872, a slight effort brought on palsy of the left arm, so that she had finally loss of power in both hands, with loss of voice. This was followed by anuria, and then by complete absence of saliva, so that for a time the mouth was absolutely dry. Meanwhile speechless, and with paralysis of all her limbs, she could only call any one by seizing the handle of a small bell in her teeth and shaking the head. After a year and a half the use of induction currents seemed to have a good effect, and she was soon able to use her hands, and to walk. At this time and for seven years the right hand swelled enormously before each menstrual flow, and at the close of the week the skin came off in large patches. In 1876, she had violent retro-spasms of the head and motor ataxia of the legs.

In 1877, she had hysterical convulsions, photophobia, a variety of pains, glossitis, with great swelling of the tongue, long attacks of coma, hysterical vomiting, and two weeks of nearly complete fasting, and spasmodic ptosis.

You will, I think, agree with me that a more miserable catalogue of ills could hardly be made out. Within a year the more active troubles have faded away, and we have before us only a weak, pale, sensitive woman, with complete loss of voice.

You will remember that this woman was at my last clinic, and that I told her she could probably learn to speak. Two days later she wrote to me that, for the first time in ten years, she had made a sound, and this is all, but in the mean while I asked her to come to my house, and there I studied her case yet more carefully; and now to-day she comes back, and I shall test the value of the theory I have formed as to her case. But, before I do this, let me say a few words as to the types of aphonia and dysphonia connected with hysteria. You will find in Cohen's excellent book, and in Ziemssen, very good accounts of this group of disorders, but I think it will admit of further study, and I, therefore, venture here to tell you about it some things which are not found in the text-books.

Hysterical loss of voice is apt to come on in long cases of hysteria without apparent cause. The voice goes and comes, is hoarse or feeble, and at last becomes reduced to a whisper, or is lost altogether for weeks or years. Then the patient has to write what she would have talked; and if, as in this girl's case, her arms be palsied for a time, only manual signs re-

17

main until the people around her learn to read those labial signs with which communication at length becomes so easy as to take away desire to make the painful effort at audible speech.

In a few cases emotion causes abrupt loss of speech power. Cohen relates such a case; I have seen several. Nor when we remember that it is through the voice-muscles that we express so many of our emotions, can we wonder that it is in the larynx that we feel the choking spasm of grief, or that here, also, intense sense of pathos, or almost any deep feeling, asserts its power by some act of muscular spasm; or that in nervous people yet graver emotional shocks result in the palsy of the organs through which we are prone to express emotion.

There are, as I have seen them clinically, at least three forms of hysteric conditions which disturb vocal utterance, and these three forms are sometimes all seen in one case, or may exist distinct. We have, first, bilateral palsy of the adductors of the vocal cords; second, disassociation of the various organs needed in phonation; third, habitual spasm, or sense of spasm, during use of the larynx in speech.

The first, or bilateral loss or lack of power in the crico-arytenoid muscles, is the common type of hysterical aphonia, and is usually found with loss of power in some of the other muscles of the larynx. If, in a case of hysteria, you have loss of voice, or suddenly the patient becomes a whisperer, you may be pretty sure that you have to deal with this form of trouble. Even if there has been a cold and sore throat, with cough, you may safely conclude that the slight local inflammation did not cause the aphonia, but acted as what I may call a hint to the hysterical condition. This caution is, I may add, the more needed because an outbreak of this form of trouble is often caused by catarrh; but this is the kind of thing we see every day in hysteria. The catarrh passes into hysteric paresis. A diarrhœa from over-eating becomes an hysterical diarrhœa; an attack of true emesis from indigestion is the parent of hysterical regurgitation, and this may last for years.

Bilateral hysteric palsy of the vocal cords may be extreme or slight, but where it is marked you will see, with the laryngoscope, that the cords do not come well together when the patient makes vowel sounds. One cord may come nearer the middle line than the other, but neither does its duty. This is an easy examination commonly, because, as a rule, hysterical people are not at all disturbed or gagged by the mirror; but this is not always so, and the patient we see to-day has a quite sensitive throat. If you find a distinct unilateral glottic palsy, you have, probably, a non-hysterical paralysis—at least I have never seen a monoplegic state of larynx which was hysterical. You would naturally suppose that aphonia and dysphagia would often be found together, but this is rare, very rare, although I can recall cases where the two disorders alternated.

The loss of voice in hysteric aphonia has some odd peculiarities, or rather exceptions: the patient cannot speak, or can only whisper with mouth or larynx so faintly as to be scarcely heard with the aid of the ear-trumpet; yet she may be able to sing well, as happened in one of Cohen's cases; or, as chanced in that of a lady whom we saw together, she may be able to speak aloud in her sleep, and then only. On these occasions the unwonted sound of her own voice would awaken her, and the disappointment which followed the next waking effort at speech was most distressing, and the emotion thus occasioned gave rise, like all emotion in such cases, to an even greater loss of what mere whispering power was left.

Many examples of these disorders are seen in pretty strong, stout, and even ruddy women, and when met with in such persons are, like all the hysterical phenomena of the nearly healthy, especially unmanageable. When hysteric aphonia is found in feeble and easily-tired women, the effort to speak or cough with an open larynx, or with weak chest muscles, gives rise to a good deal of soreness, and emphasizes that sense of painful fatigue about the pectoral region of which this class of invalids is so apt to complain. The victim of this disease is very often able to speak low, the voice breaking at times. Other and extreme cases lose the power to whisper with the larynx, and can still whisper with the mouth; and others, again, are unable to utter the faintest sound, or to laugh or cough so as to be heard at all. It must be obvious to you that, in the worst cases, we have here a dual condition, a paralysis which, though without coarse organic cause, may be lasting, and a disassociation of the motor activities of the respiratory, laryngeal, and buccal and oral muscles—parts which, by physiological construction and long habit, unite to produce voice. The two troubles are often seen together in variable degrees; or the incoördination may exist alone, there being still power to close the larynx.

We should then have the second and less well-known form of aphonia, and this it is well to study with care. The present case is a perfect example. If, while using the throat mirror, I ask her to sound the broad A, the vocal cords come together, but do not vibrate, because she is unable to use synchronously the respiratory muscles to drive air through the narrowed orifice. Of course there is no laryngeal whisper. In some of these cases, as I have seen, the patient can whistle more or less well, because for this act only the mouth and an expiratory effort are needed; but there are others who cannot execute even this simple act of coördination, and these persons would seem, therefore, to have also lost power to use vocally the lesser bellows—the mouth —in connection with the tongue and lips, so that in this case buccal whispering would also be lost, and the patient would then have what Cohen calls apsithuria, and be absolutely whisperless. I will defer speaking of the third form of dysphonia until we consider the case before us. This young woman has good power over the laryngeal muscles. I ask her to speak; she makes a great effort, but, as I found in my last examination, I cannot hear her even with an ear-trumpet. She has neither with larynx nor mouth capacity to whisper. She can whistle feebly, but whistling is not a feminine accomplishment, or she might do better. You observe that, when trying to speak, she makes extreme movements of the lips, and this is done to enable her friends to read this language of oral signs which she thus renders clear or emphatic.

17*

What I have here said well enough describes this curious condition, which seems not to have been very clearly recognized as being sometimes a state apart from paralytic conditions. I can give no explanation of the immediate causes of these singular incoördinations. Let us now test their presence. It has occurred to me that, if I could teach her how once more to use with success these disunited activities, she might regain her voice. On thinking how I could best bring this about, it seemed to me that, if I could teach her to speak only with a very full chest, I might secure an involuntary success in driving air through the larynx. I shall ask her to fill her lungs several times, and, when very full, to keep her mouth wide open, and, as she sounds or tries to sound the broad A, to breathe out violently. I aid her by myself performing the act. To her surprise, for the first time in ten years, she makes a clear, audible sound. Then, always insisting on each single letter being made with very full chest, we go over the vowels, and then try the labials, and at last words. As she leaves me she says, "Thank you." I insist that she shall not speak save with a full chest; that she must never use oral signs alone; and that she must be silent except during the lessons her sister will now give her thrice a day.

If this had been a case of glottic palsy, I should think her sudden cure was due to the emotions caused by her novel treatment, as Cohen has seen, and I also, the mere use of the throat mirror restore voice; but at her first visit here we got no result from this or from Oliver's method of manipulating the larynx, so that

I myself shall believe that the result was due to my teaching unused organs the easiest way to regain their habitual function.

Under the use of tonics, rest, and full feeding, with vocal lessons, and a continued order not to speak at other times, she has continuously improved. Whether or not she will relapse depends a good deal on her surroundings. Such cases are only too prone to fall back.

Hysterical spasm of the larynx is a phrase which I almost hesitate to use, since I cannot be absolutely sure that the disorder I shall describe is really due to this cause. There are few of us who, at some time of our lives, have not known the sensation of choking in the throat from emotion. It is a brief and unpleasant matter, and for well people a rare one, but among highly-nervous people, or hysterical women, there is a rare form of this trouble, or something allied to it, which gives rise to temporary loss or inhibition of voice. At first from emotion, worries, or without known cause, there is felt in or about the larynx a sense of momentary strangling and pain. If the person is speaking, the voice breaks, and she remains speechless, or the voice becomes shrill and then breaks. At every effort there is pain, distress referred to the larynx, and squeaky, broken tones. There is also a sense of constriction, and sometimes the œsophagus seems to share in the annoyance, and an upward gulping effort follows or accompanies the laryngeal disturbance. I have seen this group of symptoms become so frequent in one case, that at length the girl refused to speak at all. It was apt in this case to follow meals, and these were seasons of real suffering, because of the intense dysphagia, which caused her to chew every morsel for many minutes before venturing upon the task of deglutition. The meal became, therefore, a severe strain upon an already feeble constitution, and this seemed to have something to do with the more ready causation of the laryngeal disorder at these special seasons. A long course of milk and soup diet, inhalations of nitrite of amyl, and galvanization of the larynx finally relieved greatly these troubles, but there was no entire cure until a year later I succeeded in materially improving her general condition.

We have, then, laryngeal palsies usually with, sometimes without, incoördination of the chest, diaphragm, and mouth; pure incoördination without paralysis; and, lastly, a disease which seems to be a temporary spasm of the vocal muscles of the larynx, caused by effort at speech, in other words, a functional spasm.

LECTURE XII.

GASTRO-INTESTINAL DISORDERS OF HYSTERIA.

I HAVE said in these lectures very little as to the gravest of hysterical symptoms—the persistent hystero-epilepsies, and the multiple and severe contractions which Charcot and others describe. I have said little because, in my experience, and it has been very great, these terrible cases are rare in America in any class of life, and most uncommon in the lower classes, among which Charcot seems to have found his worst and most interesting cases. In this disorder, as in chorea and many other diseases, there is, I suspect, some difference between this country and Europe.

My own clinic furnishes yearly hundreds of cases of neural maladies, but while I often see examples of every type of the milder forms of hysteria, it is extremely uncommon to encounter the more severe and lasting forms of the disease.

My friend, Dr. C. K. Mills, who has charge of the extensive out-wards for incurables at the Philadelphia Hospital, writes me that his experience is similar to mine. He says: "My wards contain some cases of hysteria of long duration, but they are not numerous. As the result of some experience, both in and out of hospitals, I have come to the conclusion

that cases of grave hysteria, such as the hystero-epilepsies of Charcot, are rare in this city and country.
Spasmodic disorders, associated with hysteria, do not
seem to me to be as frequent here as abroad. Hysterical palsies are more often met with. Neuralgia,
spinal irritation, ovarian hyperæsthesia, and special
forms of mental and moral perversion are, in my experience, the more usual forms of American hysteria."
It is impossible to acquire as to a matter like this
precise statistical information, but from what I know
of the experience of other physicians in New York,
Boston, Baltimore, and Chicago, there is every reason
to believe that it does not differ from the views enter-
tained by Dr. Mills and myself. The causes of this
difference in the symptom-products of a disease so
common, and which finds in all lands and all female
human nature enough conditions favorable to its
growth, would be a somewhat interesting inquiry, but
one for which I must confess there is yet wanting
satisfactory material.

I have given in the final lesson of this volume
some general directions as to the treatment of extreme
cases of malnutrition and hysteria. I would like to
make here some remarks as to the especial difficulties
which meet us in connection with the stomach and
bowels of hysterical women. No matter whether we
treat them, as is preferable, by exercise and baths
and fresh air and tonics, or are driven in despair to
the more unnatural treatment by seclusion and rest,
we have still in all cases to feed them, and in all to
see that the bowels are kept reasonably open. The
lighter cases of hysteria which come afoot to my

clinic can give you no idea of the gigantic, almost grotesque proportions which symptoms may assume in the graver cases of hysteria, but in each and all it is nearly always some trick of the stomach or gastro-intestinal tract which soon or late baffles or perplexes us. In one case you have an apparent inability to chew; food rests in the mouth until helplessly removed by a nurse or is half passively let fall out by the patient. I have such a case now. I had to begin by admitting an interest in her failures and advising her to move the jaw with the hands, which she did do for a while until the power or the belief in the power to chew came back. Next comes the œsophagus with its troubles—at times a spasm, at times a paralytic state,· more rarely a pharyngeal anæsthesia—but in each case attention to the act of swallowing helps to embarrass it.

You will be well off if you escape this exasperating disorder in your early hysterical cases. It is most enduring, and difficult of relief. I think it curious that in my experience this trouble is rare in old hysteric cases. There are symptoms which are relatively common early in cases, others which are seen later, and are apt to last. Dysphagia one sees often in cases which are afoot.

If we fail of this annoyance, we may have to meet certain gastric disorders. One is loss of appetite, anorexia; the other is vomiting. Of this latter symptom I have already said something in a former lecture. What I now refer to is the simple regurgitation which we meet with in these cases. There is no nausea—certainly after a while none,—but the food is returned to the outer air with a gulp, and often with remarkable and painless ease.

You may think this sounds like a rather mild malady; but in reality it is one of the symptoms which, while it may haunt any stage of hysteria, is of all symptoms except multiple contractions the most enduring. I can now recall five cases of hysteria lasting from fifteen to twenty-five years. All are bed-ridden; and while four have contractions, three are in the habit of vomiting every meal; and have done this for years. One has actually grown stout under this; but she is an opium-eater, and rest with opium greatly aids the storing up of unwholesome fat. The others are at least not wasted, and you ask yourself in vain how they live upon the small amount they seem to retain. In reality there is apt to be some deception as to this. Nearly always these women assure you that they throw up all of each meal; but they are apt to go through with the matter alone or unseen, and no one takes the trouble to learn how much is really retained. I did take this trouble once, in a case of which by and by I shall say more, and learned that about one-third to one-half of the meal remained. In an hysterical girl at absolute rest this might very well answer to nourish her amply.

I put aside for the time the symptom loss of appetite, because of all of the embarrassments we meet with, this is the worst. To call this loss of appetite, anorexia, but feebly characterizes this sympton. It is rather an annihilation of appetite, a lack so complete that it seems in some cases impossible ever to eat again. Out of it grows an indisposition to eat at all, an antagonism to food, which results at last and in its worse forms in spasms on the approach of food, and thus in turn to some of those remarkable cases of survival for long periods without food, which you need not confound with the more or less successful efforts to deceive by the pretence of fasting. You will have constantly to deal with the various grades of this disorder, if you are called upon to treat hysteria. When it is merely anorexia, you may disregard it as you would the anorexia of fever, no matter how extreme it may be, and indeed the more so because it is extreme. There are some useful hints which you may keep in mind for these contingencies. Fluids can be taken when solids are inhibited by the disgust they cause, but, as regards solids themselves, if they be finely divided or put in a fluid as mincemeat in soup or rice in milk, they are sometimes taken well whilst if alone they would be rejected. I may also add that if the patient be in bed you will often be able to give solids, if the nurse herself feeds the patient, since then you get rid of at least one volitional act, and the added chance for deliberation, and consequent disgust which it affords.

Sometimes this symptom exists only at the menstrual period, or is then greatly intensified, and, as at this time the consequences due to loss of blood are in feeble women made worse by failure to eat, one of the most valuable lessons you can teach such women is the absolute need to eat, or, at least, to drink nutritive food, whether it be agreeable or not. The graver cases of self-starvation which arise out of the superlative degree of hysterical indifference to food are far more serious.

18

They result, as I have said, in the patient taking no food, and sometimes before such cases the utmost skill and the largest experience are simply impotent. Few of these cases exist without there being a certain amount of doubt as to whether or not these long fasts are really fasts, yet, as regards some of them, there can, I think, be no doubt; but in no real case has the duration of the fast reached that affirmed to have existed in examples like that of Louise Lateau.

I have seen several instances of extreme fasting, and I propose now to call your attention to two of them which possess a peculiar interest. The first one I studied with extreme care and with every possible advantage; the second came to me long after the time of fasting had passed, and although a woman to all appearances hopelessly hysterical, completely recovered. Her fast was observed by physicians as competent as Charcot and Brown-Séquard, and of it I have a very good history :—

Miss L. C.,.æt. now 38 years, had in her 18th year an unhappy love affair, and soon afterwards a fall in which she struck her back. Within a few weeks intense spinal irritation set in, for which braces and corsets were used, and, these failing, rest in bed was prescribed. The latter remedy was a fatal one, and she has never since left the bed to which a physician's orders sent her. It were tedious and useless to dwell on the wild variety of symptoms which followed, as we are dealing now with only one of them. Hysterical paralyses, anæsthesias, ischuria, anuria, polyuria, hyperæsthesias of skin, eyes, and ears, succeeded one another singly or in perplexing groups. A year or more before I first saw her, contractions of the two legs and feet began, and went on from bad to worse; while both legs to the waist were insensible to pain and changing temperatures, but still appreciated the position of a touch quite fairly well. The body was excessively wasted, the skin dry and sallow, and covered with bran-like scales of epithelium. About the sixth year of her disorder she began to have a constipation so obstinate that neither drugs nor mechanical aid was of the slightest use, and from this time for years the bowels were moved but once a month, at which time there were violent attacks of hystero-epilepsy. At or near the time when this difficulty developed itself fully, she ceased to pass water more than once a day. With the help of careful nurses, I was able to study this curious symptom which in her assumed an unusual form. During thirty-nine days her urine reached a daily average of three ounces. The specific gravity was 1040 to 1060. It was dark, and clouded with urates and crystals of oxalates and uric acid. The pulse rose to 120; the respirations to 60 or 70; and in place of the usual vomiting, which Charcot has studied so admirably and which he has shown to be vicarious and charged with urea, profuse sweats broke out, and left the skin covered with a white film in which I found large quantities of urea. Then the scene changed, and about the thirty-ninth day the sweats ceased, violent vomiting with nausea followed, and she began to drink vast quantities of water, which seemed to be absorbed with great speed, since the vomiting which took place at intervals was merely of a thick, slimy mucus. At the same time the anuria ceased, and, from passing some days no urine at all, she poured forth large amounts of limpid water, sp. gr. 1005 to 1012.

The fluid thus secreted averaged, for ten days, five to ten quarts; but the amount swallowed was equal or more in amount. By degrees this symptom faded away, and she drank less and less, and ate almost nothing; until, at the close of another month, the urine growing smaller in amount, she ceased to vomit, except when urged to take food. Her condition was then as follows: She passed six to ten ounces of urine daily, and drank, by the teaspoon, about twelve to fourteen ounces of water. She took no food at all for ten days, and then ate a few teaspoonfuls of milk, which always caused vomiting. From this time twenty days passed, during which she took no food, but had fifty to eighty drops of laudanum daily, which she never vomited. Her eyes remained closed, the least vibration or light caused agonizing cries, and every one expected to see her die at any moment. Efforts at rectal feeding or inunction of oils gave rise to horrible spasms, and in this condition day after day went by. The watch over her was rigid and faithful, and every effort even to give a teaspoonful of fluid was carefully noted. I am as sure as I can be of anything that in one month and five days she never took in all more than twenty-four ounces of milk, and the amount of water I have mentioned. Whether this almost incredible abstinence was aided by the large quantity of opium taken is, at least, difficult to say. There were, during the time in question, a large number of hysterical spasms, but, with this exception, the patient lay almost motionless. Now, as yet, we quite lack material for the determination of the nutritive needs of a body at absolute rest; so that it is hard to decide how much is needed for the mere sustenance of necessary function. I have seen a woman, weighing one hundred pounds, remain at rest in bed, and lose no weight in ten days on a diet of one pint of good milk daily.

Certainly my patient lost weight. At the close of her fast, when she began to take and retain milk in small portions, she was wasted almost to the last degree, and this has never failed to happen in such experiences as I have had of true fasting. This woman had in all three periods of abstinence, but the one I have described was by far the longest. The contractions have of late years become more and more extreme, and, as they have increased, the anæsthesia has become less, while the electro-muscular excitability of the leg-muscles has lessened. I have little doubt that the lateral columns of the cord are now in a state of advanced sclerosis.

The second case of fasting was also one of extreme interest, because abstinence was one of a series of most interesting phenomena, covering some years; and resulting, finally, in a complete restoration to health.

Miss L., of Connecticut, æt. now 28 years, went abroad after having suffered a long and severe strain on her emotions and sympathies; a strain which did not lessen, but from which she fled in despair. The results were broken sleep, great, though suppressed nervousness, but no notable functional disturbances.

18*

To keep down this sensation of nervous excitement she was accustomed to walk for hours, returning home with increasing pain and tenderness of the spine, the back of the head, and the scalp in general. The symptoms were thought grave, and were at last treated by a long blister over the spine. On removal of the blister there was a furious outbreak of weeping, general convulsions, and incessant local spasms of the extremities, which nothing checked or lessened. These conditions lasted during February and March, and were made worse by a large crop of carbuncular boils, which formed on the part where the blister had been placed. About this time, despite the sagacious care of excellent physicians, she began to eat less and less, and at last early in April, ceased to eat at all. Exaggerated hiccough set in, furious convulsions arose at every effort to feed her, and these symptoms repeated themselves six or seven times a day, sometimes without any apparent cause. Rectal feeding was given up, because it also gave rise to spasms, and there seemed nothing to do but to wait. For twenty-seven days neither liquid nor solid was swallowed. The tongue and lips became black and dry, and cracked; the lips were thin and crusted like the teeth with sordes and blood; the breath foul; the eye sunken; respiration quick and labored; the pulse 120 to 130; and speech whispered and difficult. Meanwhile, all convulsive acts ceased, and her mind seemed at times quite clear and capable. Twice her physicians were called in to see her die; but the stupor, which seemed almost as deep as death, also, in its turn, passed away.

I am unable to give details as to the state of the

secretions during all of this long fast. The bowels were, I think, moved once, and the urine ceased to be secreted after the eighteenth day.

There was some difference of sentiment in the consultation brought about by this grave condition, one great authority advising inaction until nature asked for food, which he thought would happen. Another physician who was then consulted saw in her case an example of starvation which, having reached the limits of great peril, demanded forced feeding by the stomach tube. I am positively informed that of this counsel, which it was resolved to follow, the patient knew nothing. However, at this critical moment she motioned to her physician, and in a whisper said she could now take food. Then came two weeks of careful spoon-feeding, with constant threats of repeating the old troubles when, suddenly, a general tremor set in, and the motion growing larger, became twitching, and so by a crescendo movement went on into violent convulsive acts, until despite the care of those about her she was thrown by a series of spasms from the bed to the floor, where she lay, muffled with shawls, cloaks, and pillows to save her from bruising herself, until at length chloroform brought quiet. The summer wore away with a variety of symptoms, such as partial palsies, aphonia, and mental depression. The next autumn she was removed to Liverpool, and there during the winter she had variable degrees of anorexia, and the usual miserable variety of hysterical disorders. Treatment was varied enough, but always unavailing, because no treatment could ignore food, and that was kept at the minimum on which existence is possible. Early in the next September the girl mustered courage to cross the Atlantic, and arrived in New York, suffering with a loud, incessant cough, which brought up strange quantities of glairy mucus. Emaciated to the last degree, with evening fever and morning chills, she seemed on the verge of death. when almost suddenly the cough ceased, and the starvation symptoms reappeared, but not in so disastrous a shape as had marked their appearance in Paris. After a partially successful treatment at the hands of her physician in New York, circumstances removed her from his care. Again the stomach tube was advised and declined by the family, and again days passed without food, while the convulsions, the wasting, the black tongue, the breath, which Brown-Séquard had described as an odor like that of altered fusel oil, and the shrunken belly all promised a new period of three weeks' fasting. It proved, however, less complete than before, and she gradually rallied. From this time she remained in bed for nine months, eating little and irregularly, a wretched invalid, not very thin, but not fat, with occasional spasms, great nervousness, distressed by light, by sounds, by any company which was not quite agreeable, forever alarming her friends by threatenings of a repetition of her former troubles. I somewhat reluctantly took charge of this lady early in the following spring. The most absolute seclusion and the use of skimmed-milk diet, aided by massage, slowly triumphed over her disorder, and by and by she regained control over her too emotional tendencies. The details of this treatment I have elsewhere dwelt upon. It triumphed in this case so completely as to have restored my patient to absolute health, and to social duties and engagements which had seemed to her hopelessly lost.

The same obstinacy of symptoms which attends such happily rare cases as these is also occasionally met with in regard to the function of defecation.

You will find among hysterical and also among merely feeble people several forms of difficulty associated with this function. One which is not uncommon is a feeling of great weakness after every operation. This sometimes goes so far that the patient will show clearly enough, in the pallor and the hastened heart, how real is the sudden enfeeblement thus produced. In still less common cases the patient faints after the stool is passed, and is especially apt to do so if the evacuation be loose and therefore sudden. I know of one man in quite fair health who is never without a sense of faintness at and after a passage, while a stool at all watery is sure to cause him to faint.

Naturally enough such phenomena are frequent in the class of cases we are now considering—so that it is sometimes needful to give a little stimulus before the evacuation occurs, and also to insist on the use of a bed-pan. If you can thus break up a morbid habit, or at least make this occurrence of faintness unlikely for awhile, the gradual return to full health, which, meanwhile, you are in other ways promoting, will take care of the future.

A far more formidable symptom is the indisposition of some hysteric women to make any effort towards evacuating the bowels. They will tell you that it gives them intense pain, and that they cannot exert themselves, or else they will make, or seem to make, efforts which result only in failure. At last you begin to find that medicine does not act, and is met with resistance. It does this or it does that. It gives acute pain, or it disturbs digestion; you try other aperients, and always there is some objection, while you begin to observe that, for some reason, the doses needed are large. If, now, you make a rectal examination, you may chance to find the lower bowel full of feces, or else absolutely empty, as far as your powers of local examination enable you to reach. Either there is a palsy of the bowel somewhere, or, what is practically the same thing, there is a temporary inhibition of its natural movements. Day after day goes by in vain use of enemata and drugs. You will recall my mention, in one of these lectures, of the case of an hysterical girl thus affected, and also what I have said in the present lesson as to the case of the patient first described. In her, monthly evacuation of the bowels has continued, and is now the habit of years. I recall another case in which, after prolonged treatment, I advised that the bowels should be left to regulate themselves. Three weeks went by without an operation, and, when it came, childbirth could hardly have been worse. On another occasion five weeks elapsed, and then, what is naturally not rare in such cases, diarrhœa followed the constipation; so that for months there was this alternation—diarrhœa, tenesmus, intense straining, numberless efforts daily, and then, in a day, all movement arrested, and absence of stools for weeks.

If it happens to you, in an evil hour, to have one of these cases to treat, with the additional need to treat also the difficulties with which some tender mother surrounds such a case, you are much to be pitied. I recall such an example, which I saw in consultation some years ago. It began with a spot of abdominal tenderness over the spleen. Pressure on this caused nausea and vertigo. Then we had convulsions, hysterics, coma, enormous polyuria, and, at last, among other things, constipation. The physician in charge gave me this list of the drugs given in four days—night and morning, on each day, an ounce of castor oil; at mid day and bedtime one drop of croton oil; three drops had been used in one day. The more drugs she took the more she demanded, and yet it was impossible to see that the doses given caused pain. Meanwhile, for the nurse and mother the arrangement for each evacuation was the event of the day. A long stomach-tube was carried six or seven inches up the bowel, and a half pint of olive oil injected; then followed one quart to three of flaxseed tea. During the use of the enema one person was occupied in compressing the anal opening so as to prevent the escape of fluid. This help was made necessary on account of the great relaxation of the sphincter, into which a thumb could be passed without any resistance which could be felt to arise from a muscular act. Meanwhile, the patient, while insisting on the use of more water, was shrieking with pain. The whole affair took two to four hours, and the patient was, I thought, the least exhausted of those concerned. Sometimes, their efforts gave rise to a stool; some times, there was none for a week; and, sometimes, under the wild entreaties of the patient, these trying scenes were repeated in the night, nurse and mother being aroused to assist. I endeavored to get this girl out of the control of her family, but I did not succeed; and I believe that her hysteria is now firmly established.

LECTURE XIII.

THE TREATMENT OF OBSTINATE CASES OF NERVOUS EXHAUSTION AND HYSTERIA BY SECLUSION, REST, MASSAGE, ELECTRICITY, AND FULL FEEDING.

THE lessons I have here gathered together would be incomplete, were I not to add some more detailed statement of my views as to the general treatment of the conditions out of which arise the varied phenomena of hysteria. Nothing, I think, can be more melancholy than an honest survey of the amount of good done in hysteria by the host of drugs which go to form the so-called therapeutics of this disease. In disorders where time is valuable we may find a happy resource in the famous class of antispasmodics, but as a rule they are swiftly disappearing from the apothecary's prescription files, and the physician of our day who is called upon to treat hysteria, or general nervousness or neurasthenia, wisely contents himself with a careful estimate of causes, and an effort to deal with these by patient treatment.

Perhaps no cases are more common in general practice, none more annoying, and none more dreaded than those of hysteria, in its infinite number of forms and its infinite variety of masquerade. The lighter troubles, the spasms, rigors, nervousness, and curious mental states, which haunt the times of sexual

19

changes in a woman's life, and especially her passage into womanhood, are more or less easily dealt with. A careful study of the girl's character, of her home surroundings, of the incidents of social life, which come with the development of possible passion, will be the best guide to treatment, and with the obvious indications given us by distinct physical ailments, local or general, constitute our chief resources.

But besides these every-day manifestations of hysteria, we meet in practice with a growing class of disorders in which change of social circumstances, love affairs, disappointments, and what the French call *vies manquées*, combine with physical accidents to create invalids, who unite neurasthenic states with a bewildering list of hysterical phenomena. These are the "bed cases," the broken-down and exhausted women, the pests of many households, who constitute the despair of physicians, and who furnish those annoying examples of despotic selfishness, which wreck the constitutions of nurses and devoted relatives, and in unconscious or half-conscious self-indulgence destroy the comfort of every one about them.

These are the cases of chronic hysterical invalidism which are so difficult to deal with. There must be in every country thousands of these unhappy people. They weary doctor after doctor, go hopelessly through the various cures, and at last end in therapeutic inactivity, or find a refuge in homœopathy, which promises a pill for every symptom, and leaves them at last where it found them.

It is among such cases that we meet with the strange and interesting disorders of which I have

narrated so many in these lessons,--disorders which
are to be met, not by mere symptomatic therapeutics,
but by a full and clear comprehension of underlying
causes, and by such treatment of these, whether they
be moral or physical, as shall destroy the soil in which
hysteric phenomena flourish.

You will infer from these few introductory sen-
tences that I look upon most cases of confirmed hysteria as finally dependent on physical states or defects
which may first have been directly or indirectly due
to moral causes, or to these in conjunction with vari-
ously-produced constitutional conditions. Anæmia
gives rise to lessened power of self-control, this to
emotional disturbances, and these, in turn, to loss
of appetite, out of which, if the surroundings be
favorable, come graver nutritive disorder and endless
invalidism. This is a fair sketch of an every-day
occurrence. It would be waste of time to dilate on
matters so familiar.

In grouping cases of hysteria — and remember
that I speak now of the old and complicated and
exasperating forms of this disorder—there is one
reservation which I shall have to make, and but one.
It refers to the small group of women in whom we
witness obstinate hysteria associated with a nearly
perfect state of physical health. As I recall these
cases they have usually been women in middle life,
and in easy circumstances. I know to-day of a dozen
or so of such people who are able to walk about and
to do much as they please; women in good condition,
fat and ruddy, with sound organs and good appetites,
but ever complaining of pains and aches, and liable

on the least emotional disturbance to exhibit a quaint variety of hysterical phenomena. For these women there is usually no cure, and you will treat them in vain.

We have, then, the hysterical women who are yet well enough to be able to correct the causes of their disease by exercise and fresh air; and in this class we find abundantly the cases of hysterical joints, and all the range of mild hysteric and mimetic symptoms. Once make sure that you have such people to deal with, and common-sense hygiene, enforced by a resolute will, and, when you have their confidence, some earnestly given moral advice, will be the most they will require. Let us put these aside, and we arrive at the classes with an allusion to which I began this lesson. They are the old and habitually bed-ridden, or couch-loving invalids, who are to-day, as they have long been, the despair of the best of us. What shall we do with them?

For practical purposes we may divide them coarsely into two sets—first, the nervous and hysterical woman, who is at the same time fat, but, as a rule, anæmic. The class is not a large one, nor is its anæmia very profound. As a rule, there is a look about the fatness of these women which is anything but reassuring. They are more or less feeble, not large feeders, and prone to suffer from excessive tire upon disproportionate exertion. I have elsewhere discussed[1] at length the probability of there being chemical differences between the fat of these and of more healthy people.

---

[1] Fat and Blood.   J. B. Lippincott & Co., 1877.

There is muscle and muscle, fat and fat, and it is now become more and more sure that these mysterious variations in the quality of tissues, however little we may know of their chemistry, are such important factors in health that we cannot at all afford to disregard them. I say all this, because, when you meet with women who are at once very stout, and not too notably anæmic, you may be disposed to regard them too lightly as free from suspicion of any such grave nutritive disorders as may seem to offer reasonable explanation of their nervous symptoms. Those who are very plainly pallid and flabby, fat and feeble, will, I may here say, offer, like the rest of their class, a problem not always very easy to solve. We shall, by and by, consider how they are to be dealt with.

There remains, in the second place, the larger class of nervous, and exhausted, and hysterical women who are, as a rule, weak, pallid, flabby, disfigured by acne, or at least with rough and coarse skins; poor eaters; digesting ill; incapable of exercise, and suffering from the cold extremities which lack of this, with thin blood, occasions. They lie in bed, or on sofas, hopeless and helpless, and exhibit every conceivable variety of hysteria.

It has been for some years my custom, when in these women every other plan has failed, to deal with them by a certain combination of therapeutic means which has now been securely tested by time and hundreds of successes. It has stood the criticism and won the approval of many competent physicians, who have found in it a resource where all else had failed.

As it is now seven years since I first published[1] a formal statement of this method, it seems to me that the time has come when I should say in what respect my opinions have been altered or confirmed, and what changes I would desire to suggest. I shall, therefore, give here a condensed statement of the treatment in question, and referring to my former publications for minute details, shall criticize it in the light of what, without want of modest statement, I may venture to call an enormous experience.

The treatment to which in these pages I so many times refer, consists in an effort to lift the health of patients to a higher plane by the use of seclusion, which cuts off excitement and foolish sympathy; by rest, so complete as to exclude all causes of tire; by massage, which substitutes passive exercise for exertion; and by electrical muscular excitation, which acts in a somewhat similar manner to massage, and with it by depriving rest in bed of its essential evils, leaves only its good. These means enable us to over-feed our patients, and to enable them to digest with ease large amounts of food.

I have here put first the idea of seclusion. That means separation from indulgent friends and sympathetic relatives. It is a change in the interest of every one concerned, because a chronic invalid is a slow poison in a household of loving people. It means, too, the breaking up of old habits; and it means, usually, a change of diet and personal sur-

---

[1] Rest in the Treatment of Disease. Seguin series of Lectures. Appleton & Co., New York. Fat and Blood, 1877.

roundings, because seclusion is not often to be attained at home. For nervous or hysterical people it
must be absolute; for merely feeble people, who retain the power of self-control, and who are to be put
at rest, it admits of every degree of liberality. We
should remember, however, that even if a woman be
only a tired and weak invalid, and not a very nervous
one, she must, owing to the necessities of the treatment, see daily the masseuse, the electrician, the
nurse, and the physician, so that to admit other
visitors is to make a needless call upon her growing
strength, which in these cases is sorely taxed by conversation. I do not say that seclusion is impossible
in the home of the invalid, for I have obtained it with
success many times, when my nurse was a thoroughly
good one; but the other plan of securing it by a
change of dwelling is better and far easier. Seclusion,
of course, has for its objects the cutting off of many
hurtful influences; but, above all, it means the power
of separating the invalid from some willing slave, a
mother or a sister, whose serfdom, as usual, degrades
and destroys the despot, while it ruins the slave. Like
all rules, this latter one of isolation from habitual personal relations, has its exceptions. I have had cases
nursed successfully by a mother or a sister, but I
never wish to make the experiment, because it inevitably makes heavier the doctor's task, and because it
is nearly always an experiment. Get your patient
alone with a good nurse, with some woman who is
trained, intelligent, young, and clever enough to read
aloud, and with culture enough to make her an agreeable companion. Ten years ago there were no such

nurses; to-day there are enough of them; but in
choosing a nurse, remember that if she has no tact,
or has a short temper, or is clumsy, or un-neat, you
may have your case spoiled, or be forced to change
the nurse midway in your treatment; but, at all
events, never hesitate about this. If the patient and
nurse do not agree, make a change, and, if need be,
another. I cannot enough emphasize this matter of
the nurse. Put yourself in the place of an intelligent
lady shut up for two months with a coarse woman,
whose talk and whose habits disgust, and doubly disgust, because the victim is emotional and sensitive
by nature and by habit, and you will realize the need
for care in your choice of an attendant. Mere technical
training will not answer, and I have seen an utterly
untrained woman, of good brains and tact, win successes which are sometimes denied to the best educated nurses who lacked those ever-needed moral
qualities which no training and no length of experience will give to some women.

And now, having your patient isolated and the
nurse in charge, certain grave questions arise. We
will presume that the case has been found to be suit-
able, and that the patient has come within your own
control—whether at her home or elsewhere—that her
case is new to you, and that you have decided to use
rest. The first question you will have to settle is as
to whether it be wise when using this treatment to
correct all womb troubles at once, or to wait, or to
neglect them altogether? I am guided as to these
matters by the following rules: In the case of married women, I make or. cause to be made a thorough

examination to begin with. If there be only congestive states and their consequences, I trust to the
general treatment for cure. If there be marked dis-
placements or excessive menstruation I like to correct
the one and have the uterus well searched for possible
causes of the other. Should there be grave fissures
of the neck of the womb or perineal rupture I prefer
to have these relieved at once if the patient be in a
moderately good state, but if the case be one of extreme feebleness I prefer to delay all surgical inter-
vention until the improved conditions which follow
my treatment offer a better chance of successful
mechanical interference. If the patient be a virgin,
and there seems little reason to suspect misplace-
ments, I trust again to the general treatment. If,
moreover, there be plain evidence of misplacement,
and the patient be of that temperament which makes
vaginal examinations disastrous shocks to the nervous
system, I wait patiently the result of the rest and its
aids. Then at the close of two months I like to make
an effort at local relief, in the hope that with a rein-
forced nutritive life my patient may bear the strain.
Dr. Goodell will remember cases, seen with me, in
which the patient, having retroversion, decided to
undergo no mechanical treatment, and has seemingly
become and remained well, under rest, etc., despite
the uterine trouble.

Misplaced ovaries cause in my experience a great
deal of trouble, but both Prof. Goodell and I have seen
a number of cases in which this annoying complica-
tion righted itself spontaneously during treatment by
rest. In one of these cases, .the misplacement was so

extreme and the symptoms caused by it so grave that the propriety of double ovariotomy was more than once discussed. We were pleasurably surprised as the treatment progressed to find a gradual slipping upwards of the ovaries until at last they regained their usual place. This change accompanied a remarkable gain in vigor and in flesh. I have never yet been able to make clear to myself precisely why under these circumstances the ovaries should be drawn up, but Prof. Goodell's opinion in a matter of this kind must be far better than mine, and as he thinks there is a competent physical explanation, I give his remarks in full: "The ovaries should be daily replaced by atmospheric pressure, the knee-breast posture, and the result is that they finally go up to stay up. Under the influence of the general gain in health, and the local handling of the masseuse, the organs cease to be congested. Then the increased deposit of fat in the abdominal walls, in the omental apron, and around the viscera, to say nothing of the needful fat-padding in all the pelvic nooks and crannies, increases the retentive power of the abdomen."[1]

"By its gravity the now fat-laden and overhanging wall of the abdomen tends to draw toward itself, that is to say upward, the movable wall of the pelvis. The behavior is like that of a half-filled India-rubber ball, in which bulging at one portion causes a corresponding cupping at another."

You are now ready to put your patient at rest in bed, and you will not, I trust, despise any details which

---

[1] Lesons on Gynæcology, Goodell, p. 116.

will make rest endurable and useful. You cannot always get, but you can desire to get, sunshine, an open fireplace, a well-made bed, and a lounge for change.

Rest means with me a good deal more than merely saying "Go to bed and stay there." It means care that letters bring no worrying news, that they are brief and of such kind as a nurse may read aloud. It means absence of all possible use of brain and body. It means neither reading nor writing, at least for a time, with exceptions in cases where, as is rare, there is no asthenopia. If the nurse can read to the patient, and reading be borne without fatigue, let it be used at first for only a few minutes at a time. If this wearies, then let the nurse try to cull the bits of interesting news from the papers, and as she glances over the columns talk this to the patient in place of formally reading aloud. Why this tires less than reading I do not know, but that it does so I am sure. If you are disposed to smile because I say let the nurse feed the patient, you will not, if, lying supine, you make the experiment of using your own hands in this act of feeding. Or even if seated in bed you do this, you will find that the effort is singularly tiresome. I believe I have done something to make rest fashionable among physicians as an essential in the treatment of spinal maladies, and both in them and in the treatment of neurasthenia and hysteria it is well that you clearly comprehend what it is that I mean by rest. Your trouble will be always that the patient will desire to lie on a sofa, or to make some such compromise, but in bad cases, and it is only of these I speak, all this is but mere trifling, and you had better, on the whole, make an error in the direction of a too absolute rest.

The moral uses of enforced rest are readily estimated. From a restless life of irregular hours, from hurtful sympathy and over-zealous care, the patient passes into an atmosphere of quiet, of orderly control, and under the care of a thorough nurse. The result is always at first, whatever it may be afterwards, a sense of relief, and a remarkable and often a quite abrupt disappearance of many of the nervous symptoms which had previously harassed the patient. With this first sense of ease comes the precious chance of the doctor for moral medication. He can now point out that, however hard it was with failing powers to control emotion and suppress nervousness, it is easy to do all this when the physical condition is improving. This doctrine will be aided and enforced by the nurse if a good one, and your patient will be constantly reminded that she is getting better physically, and is expected to accomplish more and more in the way of self-restraint. If she fails you praise the effort. If she succeeds you applaud the success. You are her whole audience, and this with an hysterical girl gives you great power. Why rest is of therapeutic value I have elsewhere more fully shown. It is of more use here to urge that, like all medication, it has its evil side, and that it is to the other parts of this system we must look for the means of overcoming and counteracting them. Ordinarily prolonged rest enfeebles circulation, weakens digestion, lessens appetite, and constipates the bowels. The active muscles are every one of them pumps, which subject the local blood circuits to sudden flushing, and the heart in a person at rest loses twenty beats a minute, and thus adds to the passive mischief. Moreover, the liver and the double abdominal circulation, and the moving bowels cease to have the constant stimulation which they get when we are afoot, and so in many ways damage is done. Rest, then, is, or may be, hurtful. We turn to massage and electricity for aid in correcting this. Massage, or kneading of the muscles, has been long used in Europe and the East. It is the "shampooing" of the oriental, the "lammi lammi" of the Sandwich Islander. I do not know that it has been used except by me as a systematic daily mechanical tonic. For details of just how it ought to be done, and with what caution, and how long and what are the immediate physiological effects, I must again refer to my book, on Fat and Blood. Used daily, half an hour to an hour, it is a pleasant and refreshing process, and even when, as does happen, it seems at first to tire, all of this result, soon or late, passes away.

It substitutes exercise for exertion, and does nearly all that a moderate amount of active muscular motion can do in the way of warming the limbs, increasing the blood-flow, stimulating the local circulations, and reddening the skin. It may, and should, at last, be a pretty violent influence, and, by and by, may be used in such a way as to jog the intestines like the invaluable shaking given by a rough trotting horse. To be thoroughly done it needs a trained masseuse, but any clever person, who is strong enough, may easily learn to do it; and it enables one daily to rub into

20

the skin a large amount of some nourishing oil, like that of the olive or the cocoanut. I never could see why a tonic so valuable as this should be left to assist the triumphs of the charlatan; and I feel that, in making it of easy use, I have done that which, in many ways, is valuable to the surgeon and the physician. You will meet with some difficulty in having the back kneaded when there is spinal irritation, but as to this you must be relentless; and the masseuse, by degrees approaching the sore spots, will in time come to treat them as thoroughly as any other part, and with the sure result of, by and by, lessening and destroying the local sensitiveness. In like manner the hyperæsthesias of other regions may be dealt with, and, above all, that which is sometimes a truly ovarian, and sometimes merely an abdominal surface sensitiveness, may, with time and cautious patience, be relieved or cured.

Massage is, in these cases, absolutely essential: electricity is very desirable; but we can, in many cases, do without it.

It involves the daily use of induction currents (slow interruptions) to almost every muscle which can be reached; the object being to throw each muscle into decided contraction. Finally, a mild current with rapid breaks of current is made to pass from the neck to the feet for fifteen minutes. That it is, thus used, a powerful tonic I have not the faintest doubt, and I commonly use it with massage, except where the need to save expense is of moment.

These means are employed to prevent rest from being hurtful, and to enable us to fatten and redden the patient by a methodical system of over-feeding, with the use of proper tonics. I have already said that there is some trouble in treating fat and anæmic women. You may cure them by ordinary means, but it is easiest and safest to do so by putting them at rest, and under-feeding with milk, so as, at first, materially to reduce the flesh, after which the patient may be subjected to the usual treatment by massage and the other means I have detailed. It is easy, with perfect security, to lessen the fat rapidly, if only the patient be kept in bed; otherwise, as we have too well known, it is a dangerous and difficult thing to effect. I may add that if there is much, or a very obstinate dyspepsia, it is well to begin the treatment of any case by Carel's milk treatment. It is astonishing how this simplifies matters, and how under milk, massage, and rest the whole train of nervous ills melts away in a few days; and how we are able to dispense with chloral and morphia, or habitual use of other drugs. Indeed I may add that I should be sorry, now-a-days, to treat any old case of the opium habit without these invaluable aids.[1]

In fact, if I have the least doubt, I never fail to begin in any case of treatment by rest, with milk as the sole diet; while, of course, there are also many cases where it is used only as an adjuvant, and I simply feed the patient in the ordinary manner. By some such plan the patient has the diet gradually increased, until it is common to see her take three meals as well as two quarts of milk, six to nine ounces

[1] Am. Jour. Med. Sci., Oct. 1866.

of Hoff's fluid malt, and a variable amount of raw soup between meals and at bedtime.

Iron in large doses, alcohol rarely, and cod-liver oil, by the mouth or rectum, when well borne, are to be added as indicated.

The result of two months of such treatment, in pale, bloodless, meagre, and nervous women, must be seen to be believed or duly appreciated. You have seen it here often enough to fully understand me. Each and all of the means described are to be slowly and by degrees laid aside, and then you have as carefully to get your patient up and afoot. Of late I have been in the habit of preparing for this by allowing the nurse or masseuse to exercise the patient, while in bed, with a series of slowly-executed Swedish gymnastics, which are continued in a modified form, when the patient gets up. If this be well and pleasantly managed, it is both agreeable to the patient and a valuable means of training the muscles.

The final results of all this treatment when it succeeds are to reasonably increase the bulk of the body, to improve the moral and physical tone, and to cure the anæmia. These changes are obvious in some degree early in the case, the flesh shows first in the face and the gain in blood in the pink of the finger-nail which I am apt to watch and note. I have been many times asked if these amendments or cures are permanent, and I believe I am now, after a careful review of some hundreds of cases, fully able to say that they are quite as lasting as the cures of any nutritive defects obtained in more ordinary ways. It is a plan never to be used where exercise, outdoor life, tonics, or change have not been thoroughly tested; but where these have failed it leaves us with a novel resource without which no case of broken constitution, nervousness, or old hysteria should be left to hopeless invalidism, and to a life in bed, or on a lounge. I never use it if I can do without it; but in well-chosen cases I use it, with a confidence which has become alike courageous and habitual.

INDEX

NEW MEDICAL WORKS.

WELLS ON THE EYE—New Edition. Just Ready.

A TREATISE ON DISEASES OF THE EYE. By J. SOEL-
BERG WELLS, late Professor of Ophthalmology in King's College Hospital. Third American, from the third English edition. Thoroughly revised, with copious notes and additions
by CHARLES S. BULL, M.D., Surgeon and Pathologist to the
New York Eye and Ear Infirmary. Illustrated with over 250
engravings on wood and six colored plates, together with se-
lections from the test types of Jaeger and Snellen. In one
large and very handsome octavo volume of 900 pages. Cloth,
$5 ; leather, $6 ; very handsome half Russia, raised bands,
$6.50.

THE NATIONAL DISPENSATORY.
Second Edition. Now Ready.

THE NATIONAL DISPENSATORY ; containing the Natural
History, Chemistry, Pharmacy, Actions, and Uses of Medi-
cines, including those recognized in the Pharmacopœias of the
United States, Great Britain and Germany, with numerous re-
ferences to the French Codex. By ALFRED STILLÉ, M.D.,
LL.D., Prof. of Theory and Practice of Medicine and of Clin-
ical Medicine in the University of Pennsylvania, and JOHN
M. MAISCH, Ph.D., Prof. of Mat. Med. and Bot. in Phil. Coll.
Pharmacy, Sec'y to the American Pharmaceutical Association.
Second edition, thoroughly revised, with numerous additions.
In one very handsome octavo volume of 1692 pages, with 239
illustrations. Extra cloth, $6.75 ; leather, raised bands, $7.50 ;
very handsome half Russia, raised bands and open backs, $8.25.

FOTHERGILL'S HANDBOOK OF TREATMENT.
Second Edition. Just Ready.

THE PRACTITIONER'S HANDBOOK OF TREATMENT ;
or the Principles of Therapeutics. By J. MILNER FOTHER-
GILL, M.D. Edin., M.R.C.P. Lond., Asst. Physician to the
West London Hospital, Asst. Physician to the City of London
Hospital, etc. Second edition, revised and enlarged. In one
very neat octavo volume of about 650 pages. Cloth, $4.00 ;
very handsome half Russia, $5.50.

HENRY C. LEA'S SON & CO., Philadelphia.

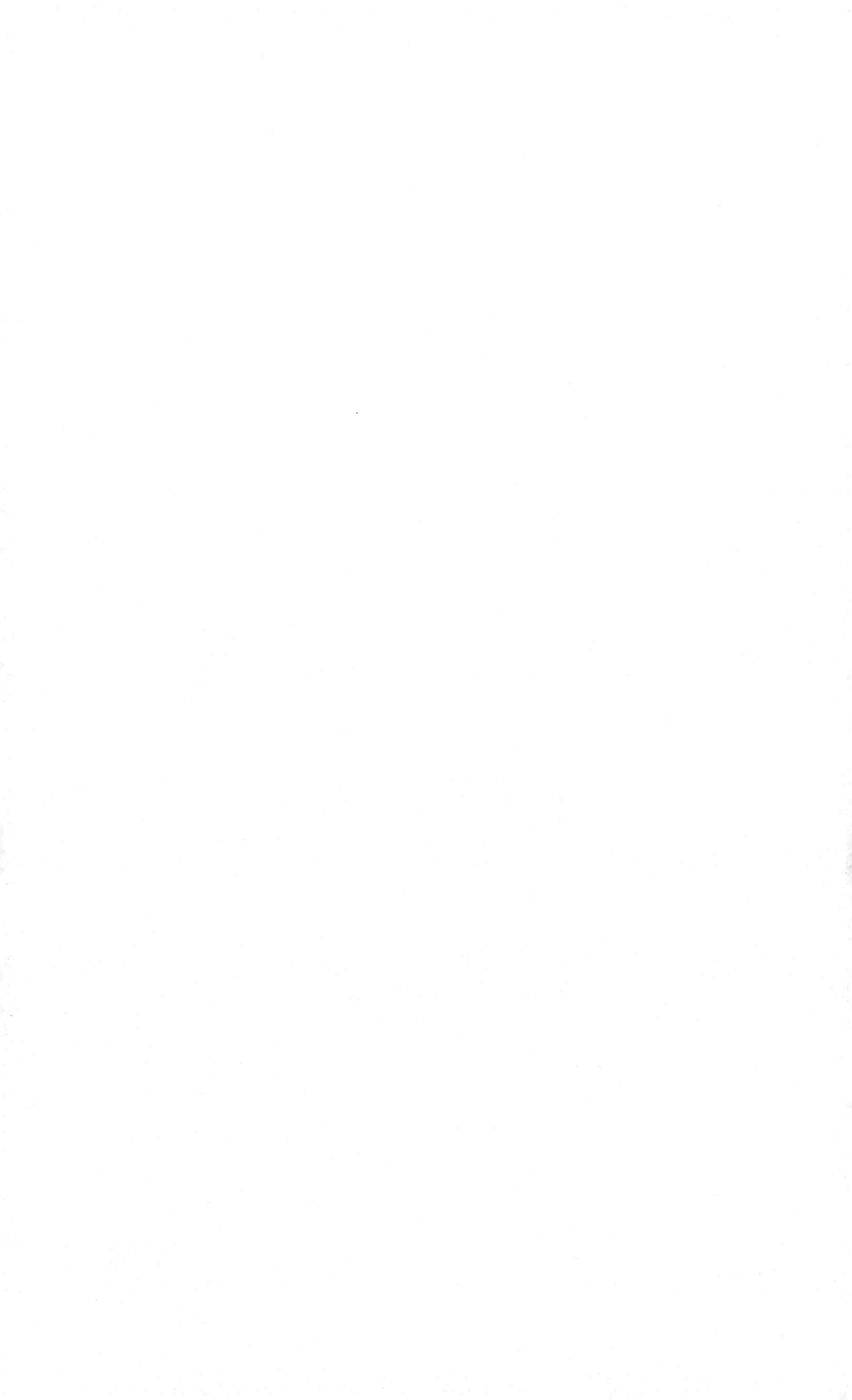

CPSIA information can be obtained at www.ICGtesting.com
Printed in the USA
BVOW11s1810091215

429866BV00019B/98/P